Weather the Storm

The heinous desire and intention of the stroke to ruin my life and destroy all I held dear was no match for my determination to fight it and recover.

by

Andrew Shaw

***A man is not measured by how he falls,
but how he gets to his feet***

AuthorHouse™ UK Ltd.
500 Avebury Boulevard
Central Milton Keynes, MK9 2BE
www.authorhouse.co.uk
Phone: 08001974150

© 2008 Andrew Shaw. All rights reserved.

No part of this book may be reproduced, stored in a retrieval system, or transmitted by any means without the written permission of the author.

First published by AuthorHouse 4/17/2008

ISBN: 978-1-4343-7503-2 (sc)

Printed in the United States of America
Bloomington, Indiana

This book is printed on acid-free paper.

Dedication

This book is dedicated to my son Tom, daughter , Amy, and my Mum, Dad, Brother and Wife. You've all influenced me more than I can express in words.

Also to all the wonderful people who have been involved in my remarkable recovery from a severe stroke including Mark Barber, Andrew Manktelow, Ralph Shelley, Jan Jolly, Jayne Gill, Ken Winfield and others to countless to mention.

The most special acknowledgement and dedication goes to Mrs Patty Shelley who cared for me and helped me as though I was special. To some I'm special but to Patty I'm one of many patients lucky enough to have benefited from her most amazing talent. Her warmth, humanity, talent and understanding have to be experienced to be understood. Eventually I realised that all Patty's patients are special to her. She cares so much for each and every one.

With admiration and love to:

Patty 'Magic Hands' Shelley. Probably the best physiotherapist in the world.

Stroke survival is both the most devastating and positive experience one can have.

Tough times don't last, tough people do

To really live you must almost die!

Foreword by Chris Dent

In preparing to write this foreword for Andy's book I thought you might be reading about his experience because you or someone very close to you has survived a stroke and is now in the recovery process. There can be recovery after a stroke – I know because I've done it myself. The recovery road is long and difficult. When I started out on the recovery road after my stroke I was told 'I'd bought a ticket for a mystery tour'. Such a comment (thanks Frank) was not and is not intended to worry or depress you but merely to offer a piece of realism. Not every stroke survivor wants to hear such as I certainly didn't.

Despite all the love and care a stroke patient needs and, hopefully, receives and the things that medical science advances allow no one can tell you how long each individual stoke recovery journey will be. I told Andy that he should be prepared to discover a lot on his journey and to take with him the love and support of his family as well as much patience. I told him to be patient and ask for the patience of those who are travelling the journey with him because such a commodity might, from the stroke survivor, be in short supply.

Bon Voyage, Andy and other stroke survivors. Please make the journey, for as daunting as it might at first appear it is worth it.

'Chris, I'm so jealous of you because your life is complete. You've got your career sorted and you have Sharon and Charlotte. You have got everything' said a colleague some years ago whilst most recently I was told by my hairdresser 'A friend of mine has had a stroke. He 's a fit, young bloke and I told him about you and he said he'd like to talk to you as he feels that if he can draw upon your experience it might help him recover.

The latter of those two conversations was my introduction to the author and how I came to be writing this foreword. Prior to our journeys I don't think either of us could have imagined seeing our words in print.

The person who told me that my life was 'sorted' thought I was fazed by nothing and that as a policeman helped other people with their problems and could deal with anything that came my way. You might imagine their horror after I, like Andy, suffered a stroke and went from someone 'with it all sorted' to a man who couldn't tie his own shoelaces and underwent a role reversal with his eight year old daughter who had to lead Daddy across the road to ensure his safety. If you are a stroke survivor or a relative of a survivor you won't need to be told how shattering the experience is but, like Andy and I, keep moving forward because you might just find that you have not just survived but can survive and prosper too. Remember, dear reader, you only complete a journey by constantly moving forward. Even an inch at a time will eventually get you there. Battle on, like Andy, and I know you can make it. We're just ordinary people really. As for Andy he's got something very special, something that many people don't have. It's not just his spirit and outlook on life it's something more but I'm not quite sure what it is. Manchester United manager Sir Alex Ferguson once said 'If I was putting Roy Keane .... [In] a one on one against anyone [he'd] win the Derby, the National , the Boat Race and anything else. It's an incredible thing he's got'. Well, I've got news for Sir Alex. Roy might just have his hands full with a certain Mr Shaw.

Contents

Dedication v
Foreword by Chris Dent ix
Introduction xv

Chapter One
Stroke! 1

Chapter Two
Far Reaching Effects 37

Chapter Three
Initial 'Care' 47

Chapter Four
Going Home 89

Chapter Five
Inspiration 97

Chapter Six
Back To Work 105

Chapter Seven
Patty Shelley 121

Chapter Eight
The Healthcare Industry 125

Chapter Nine
The World of Physiotherapy 135

Chapter Ten
Florida 141

Chapter Eleven
Exeter 147

Chapter Twelve
Two Years On 153

Chapter Thirteen
Visualisation 155

Chapter Fourteen
The World of Disability 157

Chapter Fifteen
The Final Word? 163

Chapter Sixteen
Chronology of Stroke 165

Bibliography 169

Introduction

On 13 December 2005 at the ripe age of 41 Andy underwent a resurfacing operation on his right hip but his recuperation was hindered when on December 29 he suffered a severe and debilitating stroke. At the time of these events he was holding down a difficult and demanding job at Director level with a place on the board and a sizeable income in one of the UK's largest holiday airlines. He was also immersed in a part time role as a Coach at the Notts County Football Club Centre of Excellence, working with the under 13's squad, both in the evenings and during the weekend. The stroke affected his left side causing paralysis of his arm, hand and leg in addition to his sight and speech being affected Such effects dramatically changed his life which revolved around his family, work and his love of soccer, which involved both coaching children and playing at amateur veterans level in addition to watching his favourite team - Nottingham Forest.

Chapter One

Stroke!

Leaving work on the 9th of December 2005 was a slightly odd feeling because I was facing the prospect of a hip resurfacing operation, the following week which might mean a lengthy lay off of at least a few months. Since beginning my working life in a coal mine in August 1980 I'd never had a day off due to sickness so I was breaking new ground with the thought of being in hospital or at home whilst I might otherwise have been making my contribution in the corporate world. It had been agreed that I would be off work to recover until early February 2006 and I had made all the necessary plans to ensure that our planned strategy or any work arising in my absence would be covered. I was working in a major UK airline in a job I loved as the director of risk management and safety. Very demanding, effortful and fast paced but with a wonderful team of supportive, focussed and talented people whom I loved, cared about and respected. If life is played out as a huge game of snakes and ladders then I felt I was right up near the top of the game ascending the final ladder. Every one of the wonderful team I worked with wished me luck and assured me that I would be back in the office before I knew it and I was happy to believe them not knowing that an anaconda sized slippery snake was waiting just around the corner to arrest my career progression and bring me to my knees. My right hip needed resurfacing probably because of my years as a footballer, predominantly at a low level but a footballer nevertheless as well as a competitive body builder. Such activity shouldn't have normally resulted in major surgery and I can only assume that my body was, unbeknown to me at the time, affected by misalignment such that my left hip ball and socket joint was wearing more than it should have been and certainly more than was good for my mobility. I can only speculate that as a young lad of fifteen years playing in a man's league my body wasn't ready for such combat and my bodily symmetry and alignment was damaged resulting in excessive, though initially undetected, wear upon my hip hence the need, years later, for a resurfacing operation.

On the day of the operation I was concerned that everything would go well, although I had compete faith in the surgeon, Andrew Manktelow, who was to perform the surgery, and we had been through most of the risks when I first consulted him. Oddly enough, the risk of post operative stroke was not discussed. To be honest, it wouldn't have made too much of an impact upon me anyway without a detailed explanation because stroke and its effects meant nothing to me though my grandmother died of a stroke in 1976. However, there was assurance for me in the fact that this was very much a routine operation which had been carried out on countless other people and I tried to put any lingering doubts out of my mind. My family were with me shortly before the operation and knowing my will to win and zest for life, they were confident that I would make a quick recovery and would be in the thick of the action as soon as possible. Everything went well as within a matter of hours I was back in a private room (courtesy of my health insurance) to begin the relatively short road to full mobility complete with metal hip. Working in the airline industry would be interesting from now on. I had visions of being stripped naked to pass through security scanners and still setting them off. The possibilities for comedy and confusion were endless!

Even though the room was comfortable with everything I needed I was keen to get back home quickly as I was confident that my healing would be much quicker in my own home than it would have been in unfamiliar surroundings and with people previously unknown to me. Quite soon I was able to move slowly around the room and receive visitors, most of them wanting to ply me with books, journals and magazines and fruit rather than chocolate knowing my thirst for healthy living and reading. I read very much about sport psychology as I hope to work in that field in the future.

The pain and discomfort of a surgically sliced thigh was still with me but was nothing really as each day I felt I was getting on top of my recovery and I was more than willing to push myself harder and harder, within the bounds of reasonableness and sensibility, to extend my leg movement. Life was getting back to normal as Christmas approached.

As it turned out Christmas 2005 was the usual pleasant family centred event if a little slower than normal as I still carried the reminder of the operation. Life was great! My leg was slightly sore but not painful though movement was still difficult due to the postoperative tenderness. I've never really had much time for people who exaggerate pain or illness. I'm firmly in the school of 'shut up and get on with it'. I've no time for hypochondriacs or those who wallow in self-pity or those who 'can't do it', or those who (and there are some !) like to say they're ill when they aren't ! I've never wanted people like that in my company. I'm a positive 'can do' sort of fellow and I like positive people around me. Such makes a massive difference to ones demeanour and outlook. Negativity saps whilst positivity fuels and invigorates. I felt pleased with myself that I had come through the experience and was on the mend. I thought I might even make my return to work quicker perhaps than I had promised myself. For that I was delighted as one of my Christmas presents to my soccer mad son Tom was a 3 day family break early in the New Year in Barcelona to watch the home city team take on the mighty Real Madrid – David Beckham and all. To make the trip as I had intended I needed to be fit, active and fully mobile. Unfortunately, little did I know that things were about to dramatically change thus meaning the cancellation of the trip because at around 2050hrs on Thursday 29 December 2005 as the buzz of Christmas was subsiding I decided to go to bed for the evening, meaning facing the challenge of the stairs on crutches due to the surgery two weeks previously. I managed to overcome the challenge, I always do- it's the way I am – but little did I know that perhaps the biggest challenge of my life was waiting just around the corner. I made it up the stairs and as I lay on the bed I experienced a most painful and searing headache, which was most unusual for me as I never get headaches. In fact I never get anything other than the odd snuffle! However, the head pain I was suffering was intense and something more than a run of the mill tension headache. It was, in fact, the mother of all headaches, and I immediately realised something was certainly very wrong.

I was having a stroke!

> Knowledge Nugget– Forrest Gump's momma was correct – life is like a box of chocolates – you never know what your gonna get! Think of stroke as a coffee cream – fucking horrible. Alternatively, life might be like one giant game of soccer – you never know when your gonna concede a goal!

If my life is one great big soccer match rather than a game of snakes and ladders then in soccer terms I had fallen behind!

Stroke 1 Andy Shaw 0

I looked at the bedside clock, which indicated 2100 hours. I called out to my daughter, Amy, who was wandering nearby. I wanted to say "please would you get mum and ask her if she knows where the headache tablets are" but I couldn't speak! Something came out but it was a gibberish and slurred voice alien to me as it sounded like I had consumed alcohol sufficient to render me paralytic! That couldn't be the case for a teetotal non-smoking fit young fellow like me! I suspected stoke from my limited knowledge of the condition making my diagnosis based upon slurred speech and a life side, which appeared to have simply just switched off. More than that, I became aware of diminishing sight. My vision was being switched off too. Straight ahead I could see blurred lights though everything was beginning to dim and darken. Blackness descended upon me from the side as my vision deserted me. I was going blind and I was feeling frightened. All of that in a matter of a few life changing seconds – blind, dumb and partially paralysed! As the months have passed it has become clear to me that there is nothing in life that allows suitable preparation for the battle against serious ill health and, in my case, the horrific effects that stroke can bring. Thankfully my wife acted quickly, alerting the emergency services and an ambulance arrived soon after. Had my condition not been attended to quickly only death was waiting to take me to a lost eternity. I wasn't ready for that but things come along in life whether we are ready or not. Good or bad.

In time I learned from my medical notes written after both CT (computed tomography) and MRI (magnetic resonance imaging) brain scans were conducted that I had suffered, *'quite extensive cerebral infraction (brain cell death) in the right basal ganglia region and occlusion of the M1 segment of the right middle cerebral artery consistent with thrombotic obstruction (blood clot blockage) confirming the clinical diagnosis of stroke'*. For me a lifeless left side, slurred speech, lost vision and an inability to sit up without listing to the left – I had become a weeble! - were consistent with shock, worry and anxiety. Such worry and anxiety was compounded by the apparent reluctance of any doctor, or nurse to offer positive comment about my situation. The best that could be mustered was compensatory comment such as ' You're lucky to be alive'. Oddly enough, in the few weeks immediately after the stroke, I felt I was anything but lucky although I've since changed my view. Perhaps such reluctance to comment upon my situation was borne from a lack of knowledge about the recuperative powers and workings of the brain. It would appear that the medical world hasn't made much progress in its search for knowledge about the brain such is its complexity. So exactly how do you confront a fight with body inoperability via brain failure that even the medical profession has limited understanding of? The brain is the body's software and I had suffered a software failure following a power cut. In the same way that a programme glitch might affect your home computer leaving you unable to fire up a particular programme, my own software failure prevented certain limb functions. Unfortunately for me and many thousands of other stroke sufferers there are no software engineers for the brain. An immediate fix is nice to think about but is nothing more than a utopian notion at present. I couldn't be reprogrammed or rebooted! The stroke ensured my torso; shoulder, arm, leg and foot muscles on the left side of my body would not fire up. I live in my body and it is driven by my own software system - my brain. When the software fails then so does everything that relies on it. The body needs the brain like a child needs its father and a fish needs water. My body and brain are everything I am. The mental effects of sudden bodily failure via a non-traumatic brain injury are devastating, shattering, overwhelming, destroying, demoralising and anything else you can think of. Indeed Smits and Smits Boone(1994:xv) recognise that 'suffering a stroke is one of the most severe traumas a person can survive ....' I was physically and mentally floored and devastated but one thing was certain – the battle between Stroke and Andy Shaw was well and truly on and I was on the back foot.

Stroke 2 Andy Shaw 0

It was, however, difficult to be even on the back foot with the left leg paralysed and stroke affected, the right leg surgically imobile, the left arm paralysed and stroke affected. My right arm was operating seemingly perfectly. I'd gone from four limbs to one in a few weeks. One wheel on my wagon but I'm still rolling along but in real trouble though not beaten.

Stroke 3 Andy Shaw 0

One wheel on my wagon but I'm still rolling along!

I suppose years ago heart problems were feared most due to lack of knowledge about that particular organ whereas today the brain seems to constitute the final frontier in the search for complete understanding of the human body. It's vital that progress is made to give some improved understanding of the this particular organ thus improved ability to treat people who, in the future may be stricken as I am now or worse sustain a traumatic brain injury. I look forward to the day when the medical world makes the breakthrough via stem cell research or something similar to help brain problems like stroke, alzheimers and other debilitating and horrific conditions. I do hope so because it would be wonderful if such conditions could be treated and cured or even prevented altogether. Unlike many others I haven't got a terminal illness or have been affected by a problem that leaves me without hope for recovery so I shouldn't really complain about my lot and I very rarely do. I have expectation for the future. Whether such expectation is realistic only time will tell. My zest for life is intact; I'm young and alive. I've had a severe stroke but I'm here and full of life. I didn't and don't intend to let a stroke put me down and keep me there! My inner desire to fight was intact so I'm still capable of coming back to win and I have hope.

Stroke 3 Andy Shaw 1

Knowledge Nugget– Hope can't be purchased but apart from life, love, health and inner peace it feels to me like the most precious of free gifts bestowed upon mankind. It is true that the best things in life are free and that the best things in life aren't even things, certainly not material things anyway!

In the initial stages of my condition where I lay unconscious for 72 hours my family were told, I've since learned, 'The coming hours are crucial and we'll continue to monitor him but you need to be aware that his condition is very serious and his life is in the balance. He could die and you should prepare yourself for the worst!. Whatever happened in those dark hours the scales of life and death tipped in my favour for some reason. As I look back I am surprised I lived as I have always felt, as my wife could verify, that I am destined to die young after fulfilling a purpose. I don't know why I have always felt that way about my mortality but it's always been there, as has the feeling that I am on this earth for a specific purpose. Things are becoming clearer now regarding my purpose. It might be that a higher and, as yet unknown power, decided (Don't talk to me about God! If he does exist - which is highly questionable - he's very hands off, uncaring and distant) that I would be driven enough to write this book so that I might help similarly affected people. I hope I can although selfishly I'd have preferred no stroke and no book. Strokes and their effects are fucking horrible! Why did I survive? Maybe the will of a higher power so that I might fulfil the purpose set for me. Or perhaps due to my previous lifestyle of healthy eating, no alcohol or smoking along with regular exercise. Who can say? I suppose I'll never really know beyond doubt but my money is on the latter. When I emerged from wherever I might have been journeying toward I awoke to find my family around me and their expressions and tears told me of their relief that I was back in the land of the living and consciousness. It was an emotional moment. 'Daddy! You're awake!'shrieked Amy my daughter and youngest child. After waking I immediately recalled what seemed to have been a raging battle going on over my final destiny and although I still wonder if it was a dream or something that really happened during my unconscious time. When I read Gill Hicks' account (29:2007) I realised that what might have been a dream could, quite possibly, have been a real battle over my existence or death. Gill Hicks is a survivor of the London bombings despite losing her legs

Weather the Storm

in the blast and she tells (29:2007) how 'The struggle to keep my eyes open made it increasingly difficult to deny the option of going to sleep. The 'voice' of Death was comforting, I could feel myself slipping into 'her' arms. It was getting harder and harder to resist. I knew I had to make a final decision'. Hicks' account along with my own experience has convinced me that at the point of death we move into another world. I can't say for sure - no one can – and I'm not prone to thoughts of the afterlife and the unknown but I've seen the face of death closer than most and have first hand evidence that it might not be over when it's over on earth. Having experienced what I have the fear of dying now has no hold over me. I recall a conversation between two soft, sweet and convincing voices both arguing for custodial rights. One said 'What's happened has happened and I'll take him now' whilst the other said ' No, it's not his time yet. This wasn't how he has been set. He's not due until [date, month, year] .

I'm convinced it wasn't a dream and subsequently I have no fear of death - I'm beyond all of that even though I know the exact date when my life is going to end. I'm not disturbed by that, in fact it's quite a privileged position and will help me to plan and ensure my children are in the best possible position after Dad dies. I suppose I could spend time worrying that the date is getting closer but I don't and I haven't even been tempted to total up the days I have remaining. My situation is very similar to yours. I'm going to die and so are you – the difference being that I know when I'm going and that it isn't something to be feared. I've lost one life - my pre stroke life - and will, in time, lose the post stroke life too. In the subsequent days after my return to consciousness as I began to understand what had happened to me and how I might be affected (in truth I thought I understood but until, many months later as I was living through the newly created but very real nightmare I realised I was a million miles from understanding the effects of stroke). I try to use my words carefully particularly and to say my experience has been a nightmare is true. Some people say they're 'starving' when they merely have a few hunger pangs. Having a stroke and living through its after effects is a most horrendous fucking nightmare! Some things have to be experienced to understand. I suppose rather like scoring a goal in the FA Cup Final at Wembley stadium or sinking the winning putt at the Open golf Championships or landing the punch that secures the title 'heavyweight championship of the world'. I have come to believe that stroke (the brain type not the golf type !) is one thing that can only be truly understood once experienced though I still wanted to learn of similarly affected people of my age and the outcome of their plight and to do so I asked nursing staff at the Queens Medical Centre Hospital (QMC), where I found myself, if they could help. No help was forthcoming. I asked for a book or information pack about stroke. With the exception of an explanatory leaflet entitled 'Grandpa's had a Stroke' there was nothing on offer. However, for me the offer of the leaflet did two things. Firstly, it underpinned my incorrect and ill informed view that stroke only happens to the elderly and, secondly, it was the birth of this book much like McCrumb(1998: 1) who states, 'When I was seriously ill in hospital I longed to read a book that would tell me what I might expect in convalescence and also give me something to think about'.

To my continuing disappointment and regret McCrumb's excellent account was not made available to me or even recommended. It should have been. It has been a great source of help to me and I commend it to you. I've now read it four times. His account, my wife and I have agreed, almost mirrors our experience throughout. Unlike McCrumb I don't class myself as having been seriously ill although all the stroke literature seems to point to the contrary. I went to sleep and awoke and was never in any pain with the exception of a blistering headache. Indeed, if when my end does arrive it's the result of another stroke , which killed my grandmother , I don't think that would be so bad (for me at least) as, based on my experience it seems like a relatively pain free drift off toward eternity. McCrumb's stroke left him alone and unattended upon the floor whilst I was more fortunate as my family were around me and able to expedite my access to medical care. Within ten minutes of a call to the emergency services I was carried out of my bedroom and back down the stairs into the waiting ambulance. I believe I was thinking clearly and such was my confidence in the medical profession, which has since drained away, I expected to be home in the morning unmistakably showing that my knowledge of stroke was even less than limited! Although stroke is becoming more of a threat to health in the world than other more publicised and discussed conditions, complete knowledge of its causes and effects is, it would seem, as yet incomplete.

I never felt fear or pain during my journey to the Derbyshire Royal Infirmary where I was duly placed in the care of those on the Medical Assessment Unit. When my family arrived their concerned expressions told me

I was in real trouble and I felt fear for the first time because of the pace of activity around me. 'Will I die?' I thought, as a middle aged female nurse tended me. I recall vomiting onto my shirt directly onto the embroided Nottingham Forest Football Club logo giving pleasure to the, I suspect, Derby County supporting nurse who caustically commented 'best thing for it'. Derby County is our most bitter soccer rivals and since soccer is my first love and usually very prominent in my thoughts l remember wondering if I would miss any of the New Year fixtures. As it turned out I missed them all. My desire to be there was great but I had underestimated the debilitating effects of stroke. My mind was willing but the body was anything but able. The stroke had changed my life more than I could have possibly envisaged at that time. More than that as I look back in time whist writing this I really think that the Andy Shaw who celebrated Christmas 2005 did die from stroke. I am still alive but the person that I was may have gone forever although I will fight like a lion to return to something like my former physical self. It's not all bad though as I have experienced many mental and emotional changes which, when all this is over, may have a very positive effect on my life in the long future I hope to carve out and enjoy. That said I'm not sure whether it will ever be totally over as I suspect the indelible memory marks stroke has made will be with me as long as the scar on my right hip. It's effects, however, might be long gone but the knowledge of living through the experience will always be there I suspect

> Knowledge Nugget– Life is a long game. To survive the rehabilitative journey of a stroke you have to learn to play the long game. You're unlikely to get up one morning with everything back to normal. I say 'unlikely' because I believe all things are possible!

In the long run the stroke may have helped me although at the moment it's too early to tell. I'm a more compassionate, analytical and understanding man than I was. I don't get worked up anymore about things that shouldn't really matter. If my football team loses it doesn't wreck my whole weekend now like it used to do. It no longer seems as important as it once was although I still love Nottingham Forest Football Club dearly and desperately want to see the team win every game. Furthermore I have a better understanding of and grasp upon my, and other people's, emotions, Many things are very different for me now. Most importantly, I've had the time to be with people more than my previous hectic lifestyle allowed. I've been able to spend more time with my parents and also with my wonderful children, Tom and Amy. People talk about the work /life balance and mine was well and truly imbalanced. The stroke has given me the opportunity to take a look at my life for what it really was. I have to be honest and say that pre stroke I found more time for the corporate demands I had than for my family. How could I have been so stupid? Why did I almost have to die before I realised something so obvious and important.

I've made the necessary life changes now because I've been fortunate enough to have the opportunity so to do. I now get much more pleasure feeding the ducks in my local country park than I ever did from some high powered business board discussion. The ducks like to see me and I doubt any one of the beautiful feathery creatures will try to stab me in the back or get one over on me. It's nice to feed the ducks. I've missed it!

> Knowledge nugget! – Get the work /life balance right. e.g. tipped in the favour of life. Do it now because unlike me you might not get the chance to make amends later and there are no pockets in shrouds. How many material possessions would you exchange for more time with your loved ones?

As time moved on I passed through what I considered to be the stages of grieving for my previously active self. I went through a long period of anger and resentment underpinned by a damaging 'why me ' attitude, which was undoubtedly detrimental to my recovery but such feelings were dispelled as I found myself coming to terms with what had happened. though such wasn't until over a year had passed.

Whilst many things are now different for me now, 'different' doesn't necessarily mean worse. So if you are a stroke survivor don't despair. And be a survivor rather than a victim. The key word is 'survivor' and there is nothing greater than life itself. Nevertheless, immediately after the stroke I did spend many hours wondering about how life would be for me post stroke. I needed hope and my unremitting search for help produced fruit in the form of Andy McCann (2006:85) who, in his excellent book 'Stroke Survivor', explains far better than I could informing 'you had better consider how you were pre-stroke is no longer the norm for you. Enjoy the memories and make the most of what the new norm may be. In time they may overlap more than you think they could right now. Just get on with life'. I've received excellent advice from many people throughout my life but McCann's offering really resonated and underpinned my own vision of how things might look in the future. His advice has proved correct and it can for you too !

Stroke 3 Andy Shaw 2

I hope my account, punctuated with what I have termed knowledge nuggets, can give you some useful pointers to help you get on the recovery road and maximise your rehabilitation. I don't profess to be a medical expert – there would appear to be no such person (with the exception of one lady – I'll come to her later) in the world of stroke and stroke recovery anyway - but I can report from the faraway land of 'stroke survivor' and tell you how I negotiated the terrain in my attempt to return to my previous habitat of normal life.

I know life is different for me now but change is not always bad and I think the stroke has made me a better person although life is not as good as it was. You might notice that I refer to the stroke which affected me as 'the stroke' and such is for a very definite reason. Some of the hospitalised fellow stroke patients often talked in terms of 'my stroke' and medical staff oftcn ask 'whcn did you have 'your stroke?' as though it was some sort of prized possession. Fuck that ! It will never be 'my stroke' because I didn't want the fucker. I say 'my son' and 'my daughter' because I wanted them and I want them to be part of me. I'm proud of them. I'll be damned if if I'm going to talk about stroke as some sort of badge of honour. To me stroke is like the most wicked of imposters. Who wants it ?.... No one does so ' my stroke ?' Never! I was always quick to correct those who wanted to term it 'your stroke'   Strokes are killers for many but I am here and for that I have to be grateful. My wife is not a widow, my parents still have two sons, my brother still has a brother, my children still have 'Dad' and I'm still called 'Dad' because despite a functionally useless left arm and hand along with a dodgy left foot, an ungainly awkward gait and shattered self confidence they still see me as, and call me, 'Dad'. I'm still me!

Like McCrumb, I too wanted to write my account to help stroke sufferers, particularly those stricken at a relatively young age as both he and I were. I began this book thinking that I might be able to help stroke survivors and their families. I also thought it might be therapeutic for me and insightful for those dealing with stroke and practicing in the medical profession. I think it is reasonable to assume that you are reading this because you have been touched by stroke in some way. As I penned my account I hoped to fulfil the following aims for you the reader;
- What I experienced soon after the onset of stroke
- How I negotiated my way through the hospital stay
- And what happened once I was home and preparing to return to work.

Finally, I wanted to give you an idea of
- What happened in the 'end' because you, like I did myself, perhaps want to know 'Can I ever recover from this?' and 'what will life be like from now on? And 'What will be my physical condition?'

Perhaps you're impatient, as I was, to get the answer to the final point and I understand that completely so here goes! As I approach the second 'birthday' of the stroke you can be assured that, in my case, things have improved daily although sometimes it is, to me, hardly noticeable. It's rather like dieting. One wonders whether ones efforts are noticeable until you happen upon someone you haven't seen for a while who comments how well you look having lost a few pounds when you can't really tell yourself.

> Knowledge Nugget- I found that my physical improvements were hard to notice. Although they were significant to others they were, at times hardly detectable to me. I should have been recorded on video camera so I could look back at where I was. I know the evidence would have both been clear to see and a huge boost to look back upon. Record your progress !

As I write my account I'm nearly two years on from that fateful and life changing night and people constantly tell me how much better I look and how my walking is improving. I'm walking quite well now and whilst my gait is not too pretty to look at I'm getting around, my left arm is moving far better than it was, bending at the elbow and flexing to a small degree from the wrist. My hand will make a grip but won't yet release. One day it will I've decided. And I'm driving again (albeit an automatic car is all I can manage at the moment). I got back to work. I'm doing fine. I realise that every stroke and its cause is different and, therefore, each level of recovery differs. Stroke recovery is not a race, there are definitely good days and bad days and one thing is for certain – there will be setbacks and days of doubt. When doubts and setbacks came along for me I often thought of Dee Groberg's words in her excellent poem, 'The Race' which I first came across many years ago.

"Quit, give up, you're beaten!"
They shout at me and plead.
"There's just too much against you now.
This time you can't succeed."

And as I start to hang my head
In front of failure's face,
My downward fall is broken by
The memory of a race.

And hope refills my weakened will
As I recall that scene,
For just the thought of that short race
Rejuvenates my being.

A child's race, young boys, young men
How I remember well,
Excitement sure! But also fear.
It wasn't hard to tell.

They all lined up so full of hope
Each thought to win the race,
Or tie for 1st or if not that
At least take 2nd place.

And fathers watched from off the sides
Each cheering for his son,
And each boy hoped to show his Dad
That he would be the one.

The whistle blew and off they went
Young hearts and hopes afire
To win to be the hero there
Was each young boys desire.

And one boy in particular
Whose Dad was in the crowd
Was running near the lead and thought,
"My Dad will be so proud!"

But as he speeded down the field
Across a shallow dip,
The little boy who thought to win
Lost his step and slipped.

Trying hard to catch himself
His hands flew out to brace
Amid the laughter of the crowd
He fell flat on his face.

Andrew Shaw

So down he fell and with him hope
He couldn't win it now...
Embarrassed, sad he only wished
To disappear somehow.

But as he fell his Dad stood up
And showed his anxious face
Which to the boy so clearly said:
"Get up and win the race!"

He quickly rose, no damage done,
Behind a bit, that's all
And ran with all his mind and might
To make up for his fall.

So anxious to restore himself
To catch up and to win.
His mind went faster than his legs
He slipped and fell again.

He wished that he had quit before
With only one disgrace,
"I'm hopeless as a runner now.
I shouldn't try to race."

But in the laughing crowd he searched
and found his Father's face,
that steady look that said again,
"Get up and win the race!"

Weather the Storm

So up he jumped to try again
Ten yards behind the last,
"If I'm going to gain those yards," he thought,
"I've got to move real fast!"

Exerting everything he had
He regained eight or ten,
But trying so hard to catch the lead
He slipped and fell again!

Defeat! He lay there silently
A tear dropped from his eye.
"There's no sense running anymore
Three strikes; I'm out; why try!"

The will to rise had disappeared
All hope had fled away;
So far behind, so error-prone:
A loser all the way.

"I've lost so what's the use?" He thought
"I'll live with my disgrace."
But then he thought about his Dad
Who soon he'd have to face.

"Get up" an echo sounded low
"Get up and take your place,
You were not meant for failure here,
Get up and win the race!"

Andrew Shaw

"With borrowed will, Get up" It said,
"You haven't lost at all,
For winning is no more than this
To rise each time you fall."

So up he rose to run once more
And with a new commit,
He resolved that win or lose
At least he wouldn't quit.

So far behind the others now
The most he'd ever been,
Still he gave it all he had
And ran as though to win.

Three times he'd fallen stumbling
Three times he rose again,
Too far behind to hope to win
He still ran to the end.

They cheered the winning runner
As he crossed the line 1st place,
Head high, and proud and happy
No falling, no disgrace.

But when the fallen youngster
Crossed the line last place,
The crowd gave him the greater cheer
For finishing the race.

And even though he came in last
With head bowed low, unproud,
You would have thought he'd won the race
To listen to the crowd.

And to his Dad he sadly said,
"I didn't do so well,"
"To me you won!" his Father said,
"You rose each time you fell."

And now when things seem dark and hard
And difficult to face,
The memory of that little boy
Helps me in my race.

For all of life is like that race
With ups and downs and all,
And all you have to do to win
Is rise each time you fall.

"Quit, Give up, you're beaten."
They still shout in my face,
But another voice within me says,
"Get up and win the race.

    Winston Churchill was a little more succinct but less creative than Dee when he advised 'When you're going through hell, keep going'. Good advice I'm sure! As for me I never quit.

> Knowledge Nugget– stroke recovery is like dieting and 'The Race'. Set your mind to it and employ all the willpower you can muster and it can be done. Arise from your fall – keep going no matter what. Inner strength and determination is key. We really are measured not by how we fall but by how we get to our feet. The world has no time for self pity. Importantly we measure ourselves and to be satisfied with ones own self is critical. Self esteem influences mood and self esteem must be kept intact by positive action and contentment with one's behaviour and deeds.

Me at the Wembley Arena in 1994 competing in the Mr. Britain bodybuilding contest where I finished a creditable 5th in my weight class. I wasn't satisfied with my placing but was content in the knowledge that I had given my all to be in the best possible condition. As far as I was concerned 5th was nowhere and I see 2nd place merely as top of the losers as taught to me by my friend Humphrey Walters. A few years earlier I had won the Mr UK title which gave me immense satisfaction.

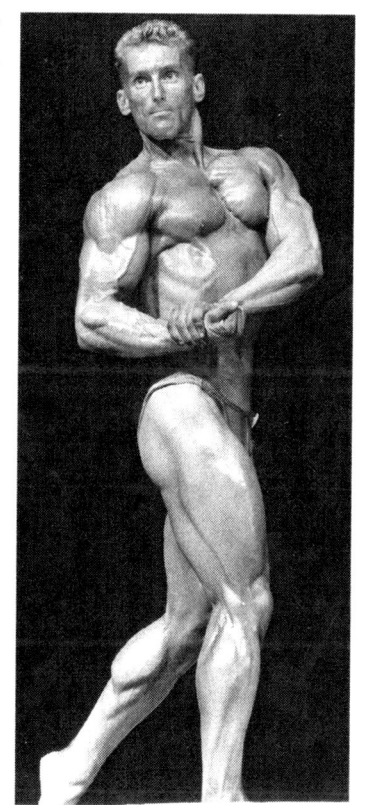

I look forward to the day when I can return to regular workouts. The stroke put an immediate stop to, amongst other things, my fitness programme, which I loved to do despite a troublesome right hip. After an intense workout I always felt rejuvenated, alive and ready to do my best in the working day. I felt that I had developed a fantastic physique by simply training as hard as was possible, nourishing and hydrating my body to optimum level whilst also using the power of the mind via visualisation techniques to vision how I wanted to look.

Here I am pictured (centre) at the Advanced Bobath physiotherapy course in Exeter in September 2007. To my right is Louise (Lou) McBarnet a member of the Stoke Madeville Hospital Stroke Rehabilitation Unit. Yoshihide (Yoshi) Hokari a Japanese student in physiotherapy working under the guidance of the wonderful Patty Shelley is on my left. Both Yoshi and Lou are magnificent practitioners. They set to work on me during the practical sessions of the course. I made dramatic gains in my physical condition during the week because of their efforts and skill.

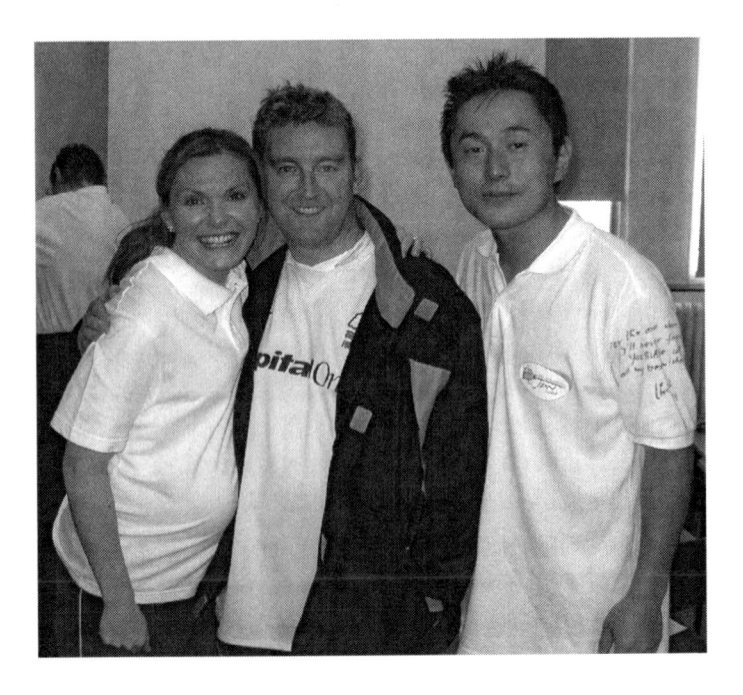

I'm pictured here having just received my Master of Science Degree in Risk, Crisis and Disaster Management after almost three years of distance learning study at Leicester University's Scarman Centre. I don't feel that I've ever finished studying and I hope to do further qualifications in future. Perhaps even in physiotherapy so that I may help other stroke victims. I'm particularly keen to look into sport psychology and such may yet be part of my future.

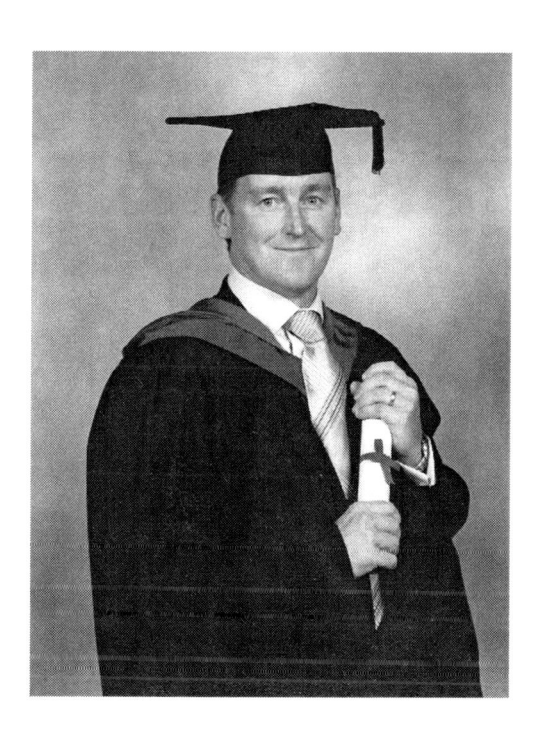

Here I am in June 2007, at the awards evening of the Nottinghamshire Football Association pictured with two of the England women's football team having been nominated for Coach of the Year. My left arm is showing signs of the effects of the stroke. I was delighted not to win because I felt that my nomination was based on the fact that I was disabled but still carried on with my coaching duties. I don't want nominating for being disabled. If I was going to win I only wanted it to be for my skill as a soccer coach. I think a disability should afford consideration and genuine heartfelt help rather than pity. I don't want anything that I haven't really earned.

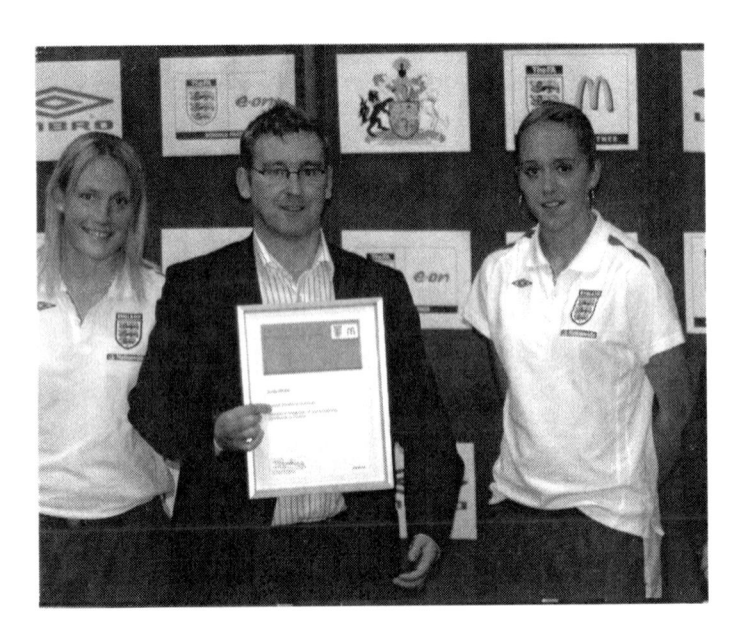

Weather the Storm

Until discovering Robert McCrumb's book I had nothing except time-restricted nurses to whom I directed my questions. I was 'contained' rather than 'attended to' on a general ward at the QMC thus knowledge of stroke seemed to be no more than, well, 'general' and if they were anything like me they were surprised that a fit 41 year old was diagnosed as such. At that time I thought of stroke in the same context as crown green bowls!

You perhaps don't think about or personally experience either unless you're of a certain age!

However I was completely mistaken about the age issue because stroke is, sadly, now affecting more young people than ever before. Rowlands (2006:06) tells us that ' …. about a quarter of strokes occur in people under 65 years old. This amounts to 25,000 people per year'

I don't know why. Maybe the pace of life, fast food, eating 'on the hoof' etc? Stress? Who can say? Like the medical profession I don't know why it is. I do know that it's very sad and unfair but one thing patently obvious to me now is that life isn't fair. There seem to be no rules regarding who is affected by ill health and other debilitating conditions.

If you're reading this to learn more about stroke and have been fortunate enough not to have a stroke yourself, let me tell you this! Do everything you can to avoid having one. The anomalous issue for me was pointed out by a friend and fellow football coach, Gary Atkin, who although very much a brusque and 'no nonsense' man has a mysterious ability to spot a situation and sum it up in a few words – that's probably why he's such a good soccer coach as he identifies and clarifies so well. He asserted his belief that the stereotypical stroke victim is advised to revise their diet to reduce cholesterol, to stop smoking and drinking and to take some exercise. Of course, that's not true of every stroke victim, including myself, but the aforementioned are classic risk factors, which accumulate over a period of years. I ate healthily, exercised strenuously on a daily basis and I didn't smoke or drink. That's how I chose to live my life yet I still succumbed to stroke, which is the most horrendous affliction I can imagine although I realise that there are certainly worse illnesses affecting people the world over every day. My cousin's husband, Alan Bacon, had a massive heart attack a number of years ago and, like myself, survived his encounter but told me recently 'When I came round from my heart attack I was able to walk, sit up, talk and use my limbs. I was truly frightened by the attack but feel that its after effects are nothing like those of stroke'. Alan's words highlight the devastation of a stroke though I wouldn't swap places with a terminally ill person and I can't begin to imagine how such a person or their families may feel. Compared to many in this world my plight, I realise, is negligible and trifling. I can't imagine how, for example, one might cope with a disease such as Motor Neurone. Similarly I don't think the effects of stroke can be understood unless experienced. They can be described but not truly understood. People often take their health for granted and trite statements about health being the most important thing are often heard. Such statements are easy to roll off the tongue but, it seems, are seldom really and truly appreciated when uttered by those enjoying good health. Indeed, it might be argued that one is, perhaps, usually in good health when making such utterances. I've been close to death and really know and understand the true value of life and good health. It's more than thinking you know the value of your health. I really do know and it's beyond all else.

> Knowledge Nugget for the healthy – every day that you are free of the devastation of serious illness is precious. Make the most of it and try to keep things in perspective. Some things are important and some aren't. Look after your body like a precious and valued friend. Don't just use it to get around! Abusing your body can take two forms – what you put into it or what you take out of it.

If you are healthy, then you will probably dismiss my 'nugget' for the healthy because ill health seems a million miles away or more accurately if you're my age, perhaps twenty, thirty, forty or fifty years away. You're probably taking it for granted right now and why on earth should you consider how ill health would affect you? I never did so it would be pious of me to suggest you should. As I write this I'm many months down the line post stoke and still consider my mortality only on rare occasions when thinking back to how things might have been. I was 72 hours away from checking out for good but I made it.

Prior to my devastating 'illness' I had not really been touched, either directly or indirectly, by serious illness or death. Surely that's the way it should be at my relatively young age. Issues of mortality seldom come to the fore and when they do it might be through the loss of a parent or grandparent. I've only ever been to two funerals. It never occurred to me that the third might be my own! It very nearly was! Aside from one of life's tragedies, a fit forty something might not even have occasion to question their 'invincibility' and mortality. In some cases there may be a subconscious belief that life will go on and on even though we know really it won't, but we do tend to think that fitness and certainly ablebodiedness will be forever in our gift. Death is a certainty for all of us and we all know it regardless of how far away it seems and how rarely we consider it. As for immobility and paralysis we just don't consider that we might be affected by it except for an accident or something of that nature. But we still don't think we'll be affected by it and there's a fair chance that we won't. But there are no guarantees as Gill Hicks will testify. I, for one, was wrong and 'It could be you' as the National lottery strap line expounds. I don't have the statistical information but why would it be you? However it's just as relevant to ask 'Why not me?' Stoke is now affecting more young people than ever before. It only takes a few seconds and whammo! Everything changes. It would seem that we all have the ticking bomb in our heads waiting to go off. Sometimes the bomb goes off early, sometimes later in life and sometimes not at all. According to the actor Kirk Douglas (2002: 5) 'Brain Attacks *(strokes)* are the third leading cause of death in America. Every minute someone in the United States has a stroke. That means more than 700,000 people each year. While you read this page, two more people will have a stroke. Thirty per cent of those who suffer strokes are under the age of sixty-five ....'. By my calculations that's something in the region of a quarter of a million 'youngsters' or people around my sort of age.

It's just not fair! Life can be going so well until, often without warning, everything changes. I thought, if only fleetingly, that I had it all and compared to many I did. I had an excellent sometimes mildly extravagant lifestyle and for that I am not ashamed. Everything I have has been as a result of the hard work I have put in and sheer effort, desire and willpower to achieve. I don't think I am naturally talented at anything but what I lack in talent I have made up for in a hunger and inner drive to do well and succeed. I never took stock about what a fantastic life I was leading comprising a healthy son and daughter, a beautiful wife, magnificent parents, a wonderful brother who loves me as much as I love him, a professionally rewarding and very well paid job, foreign travel, leisure activity, a nice home, many friends, my independence and health. I can't imagine it being better than that and never once did I think 'this can't go on- it's too good ' and indeed, why would I question something that wasn't broken? I have been fortunate that I have few regrets about my 'previous' life. (I have a new 'post stroke' life now. Things are different but they're okay. Not entirely as I'd like but okay nevertheless). I was sailing along upon the ocean of life in virtual millpond conditions when suddenly and unexpectedly I was holed below the water line. We know that life can be stormy and occasionally we hit choppy waters or even rough seas. We might even get smashed against the rocks but what makes us the individuals we are is how we deal with the storm when it comes. I'm going to weather mine. The other option is to sink to the bottom and die or fade away without a fight. I can't do that. My personality, which the stroke did not rob me of, won't allow it and I owe it to my family and friends to show them they're worth battling for and that what we once had together is worthy of my best efforts to recover.

I prefer to think my ship has been temporarily grounded and I'm tying hard to shoulder it back into the water.

My peaceful existence was threatened if not destroyed on 29 December 2005. A post operative blood clot had formed and travelled into to my brain, as I lay blissfully, albeit momentarily, ignorant thinking I just had a shocker of a headache. As I did so my young son, Tom, had entered the room and although I felt incredibly tired and lifeless just wanting to drift off to sleep, unconsciousness or whatever place I was heading for (the bottom of my ocean?), Tom urged me to keep my eyes open and stay in touch with him. I suspect he saw my droopy face, heard my alien voice and was doing the only thing he could think of to ensure Dad was communicating thus alive. Equally Tom knew something was very wrong and yet I tried to tell him via slurred speech from a paralysis stricken and droopy face I was fine, even though, quite clearly I was not and I knew it too. Foremost in my thoughts was to ensure Tom didn't become distressed. Well, I'm Dad and that's part of my role. My children's welfare comes before mine regardless of what's happening. Always has, always will.

> Knowledge nugget!- don't underestimate the effect of your ill-health on others. Understand that the spectre of ill health will profoundly affect all who love you. They may not be stricken with the illness as you are but they will be stricken nevertheless.

Chapter Two

Far Reaching Effects

My research into stroke and its effects has uncovered some startling revelations, facts and surprising data. I had some quite amazing changes and effects myself but was astounded to read about Tommy Mc Hugh as reported by Knight (Yours magazine July 07: 26) who reports 'Tommy …. is a Liverpool builder whose genius has baffled doctors world wide. Before he suffered a serious stroke in 2001 the 57 year old had never painted a picture in his adult life. But since the near fatal brain injury he has become a prolific artist'. Prior to the stroke I would have found Tommy's story incredible and difficult to believe though now it seems to be completely understandable that a brain injury, whether traumatic or non – traumatic, will result in some sort of change. I suffered some terrible physical changes but I still can't fucking paint or play the piano.

In fact , I can't claim to be able to be more creative or gifted in any area.

I'm lucky, I suppose, despite having a stroke! It could have been 'lights out' for me. It nearly was but not quite. It's important, having survived stroke, not to let its devastating effects destroy you and everything you hold dear. I have undergone some significant changes nevertheless. Interestingly my sex drive has gone through the roof and I seem to want to fulfil this increased 'desire' countless times throughout the day. Of course, unfortunately, the opportunity to fulfil the desire is not so prevalent as the desire itself ! I understand that some stroke sufferers become impotent which must be hard ! (pardon the pun) I'm at the other end of that particular scale which is favourable but I'd much prefer to be where I used to be and stroke free. Of course the other significant change is having knowledge of my date of death (assuming such wasn't just a vivid imaginary stroke induced, sub conscious dream) It didn't seem like that to me and I'm sure it wasn't. I had other physical effects that I can only put down to a change in my brain. My facial hair now grows at an incredible rate. In years gone by the growth of a beard would have been a two week project whereas now it's only a few days before I'm thick with whiskers.

I've also noticed that when I need the lavatory to urinate I need it and quick. No longer is it a steady build up of pressure to the point where I think "I'll have to go soon'. Now it's a case of 'I need to go NOW' without the previous steady build up of pressure and increased need.

Other effects have become manifest in relationships and my own feelings and thoughts. I've experienced the stages of grief in the following form:

Denial: This can't be happening to me - I'm young and fit."

Weather the Storm

Anger: "Why me? It's not fair!" Strangely at this stage I didn't look for anyone to blame for my plight. I was able to rationalise pretty well and this ability helped me whilst in the anger stage. And, wow, was I angry? I certainly was but mainly at me for being so hateful to anyone and everyone. I wasn't very keen on me most of the time.

Bargaining: I had nothing to bargain with. I was alive and grateful so I should be happy with my lot

Depression: "I'm so sad, why bother with anything – will I ever recover?"

Acceptance: This is how it is for me now so I just have to get on with it and I trust in myself that it's going to be OK.

> Knowledge nugget!- When life is bad it is still good. When life is good it is absolutely great. If you survived your stroke, that's the first hurdle over. You're alive! Life is precious – look after it and don't waste it.

I considered knowledge about my recuperation to be important and because I didn't know what to expect I used up far too much recuperative energy wondering and worrying about what might become of me.

> Knowledge nugget! - One day of worry will not add a minute to your life.

Andrew Shaw

> Knowledge nugget! - Worry may, though, be the start of finding wisdom.

I've had my fair share of injuries as an active sportsman but, of course, never a brain injury. Indeed if I'd damaged ankle ligaments, as I have in the past, I could, of course, accept and quickly come to terms with the situation but I hadn't sustained an injury with which I was familiar or ever expected. More to the point I had no knowledge of similar events and the subsequent recuperation programme. I did not know what was to become of me. Should I expect complete recovery, partial, minimal or what? Will I be forever disabled?

I worried about my recuperation and how I might progress even though I did try not to worry about things that I couldn't influence. In the scheme of things some things are important and some aren't' which I consider to be more ably explained in the speech made by Brian Bryson, also referenced by Andy McCann in his excellent book 'Stroke Survivor' which I commend to you as an informative read. I read Andy's book with interest and found it difficult to put down, probably because the stroke stopped me being able to release the grip made by my left hand! My newly damaged brain would not fire the finger extensor muscles!

Bryson asserted:

Imagine life as a game in which you are juggling some five balls in the air. You name them - work, family, health,

Weather the Storm

friends and spirit ... and you're keeping all of these in the air.

You will soon understand that work is a rubber ball. If you drop it, it will bounce back. But the other four balls - family, health, friends and spirit - are made of glass. If you drop one of these, they will be irrevocably scuffed, marked, nicked, damaged or even shattered. They will never be the same. You must understand that and strive for balance in your life.

How?

Don't undermine your worth by comparing yourself with others. It is because we are different that each of us is special. Don't set your goals by what other people deem important. Only you know what is best for you.

Don't take for granted the things closest to your heart. Cling to them as you would your life, for without them, life is meaningless.

Don't let your life slip through your fingers by living in the past or for the future. By living your life one day at a time, you live all the days of your life.

Don't give up when you still have something to give. Nothing is really over until the moment you stop trying.

Don't be afraid to admit that you are less than perfect. It is this fragile thread that binds us to each together.

Don't be afraid to encounter risks. It is by taking chances that we learn how to be brave.

Don't shut love out of your life by saying it's impossible to find time. The quickest way to receive love is to give; the fastest way to lose love is to hold it too tightly; and the best way to keep love is to give it wings!

Don't run through life so fast that you forget not only where you've been, but also where you are going.

Don't forget, a person's greatest emotional need is to feel appreciated.

Don't be afraid to learn. Knowledge is weightless, a treasure you can always carry easily.

Don't use time or words carelessly. Neither can be retrieved. Life is not a race, but a journey to be savoured each step of the way...

Bryson's speech, for me, brings a feeling of prioritisation to everyday living. As a result of the stroke I now feel I have a real understanding of what life is about, what is important and what isn't.

Friends are important and my experience of serious illness has showed me that you really do find out a lot about oneself and others. Some friends came to the fore and visited or called me regularly thus helping lift my mood and keep me buoyant, whilst others, most disappointingly, I never saw from one month to the next.

I was disappointed rather than upset and have to examine why one of my closest friends dropped me like a hot potato. Perhaps I was not easy to be around and wasn't the same fellow that I used to be although I always tried to be as upbeat as I could.

> Knowledge nugget!- I appreciate a depressive state dictates one's mood and is hard to change but try to be 'Tigger rather than Eeyore' if you can. Bouncy, bubbly and bright helps recovery rather than downcast and dour.

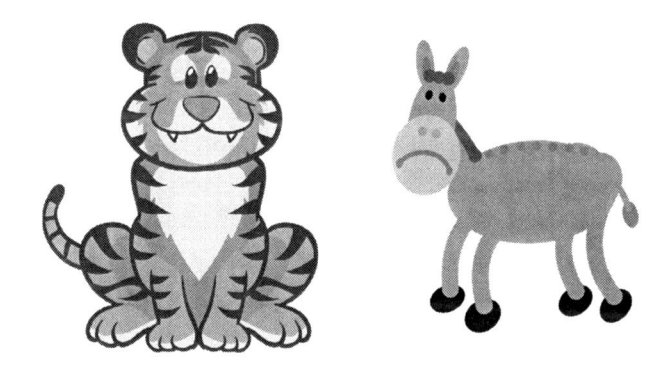

Perhaps the new Andy was difficult for my friend to accept. We used to be team mates in a Sunday evening veteran's 5 a side football league so to see me in a wheel chair in the weeks and months immediately after the stroke must have been hard for him to handle although I'll wager he wouldn't have wanted to swap his position for mine. It's strange to think that a few years ago, my wife, Lisa, and I had considered moving to America where I would have built myself a career as a ladies soccer coach. We opted against it because we didn't want to leave behind our home, parents and the friends we loved so much. Ironically, one couple who were prominent in our decision making were the couple who became lost to us as we worked our way through the effects of stroke. We understood that although our world had slowed and almost stopped others were still racing along at the usual unforgiving pace with little time for anything other than the rat race. Other friends were magnificent in their understanding and handling of the situation. I was so grateful to see many of my friends particularly my dearest friend Mark Barber along with John Matthews, John Gilbertson and Dave Smitham . These guys were really helpful and thoughtful. Sometimes it is forgotten that men can be sensitive, caring and understanding souls or am I just lucky to have friends like those? Just a telephone call from one of them was enough. They are all big strong men but they care and have sensitivity which I'd not really seen in them previously. Their kindness and thoughtfulness has made me love them even more than I did previously. Mark makes me laugh and his weekly visits to my home once I was out of hospital were of immense value. Laughter is a medicine and Mark always provides bucket loads of it. He's a natural comedian. He has been more influential in my recovery than he perhaps realises and when he and his wife Traci agreed to take a family holiday with us in Florida planned for July 2007 it was a great boost. That they agreed to come with us gave me a tremendous fillip as it showed me they had confidence in my ability to fight the effects of stroke, to be well enough to travel abroad and be good company for them. Moreover it gave me something to look forward to as

Florida, with its theme parks, natural beauty, wildlife and other attractions, is, perhaps, the most fun place in the world. Apart from Looe in Cornwall, England, Florida is my most favourite place to be and the promise of a holiday there with the Barbers was something I so desperately wanted and moreover I needed it to look forward to and, most importantly, so did my family.

Despite my love for Florida and the USA I fully intend to visit Looe again or maybe even settle there in the future. My next visit will comprise hiring a fishing boat and sailing out into the English Channel to have a relaxing day doing nothing but drinking tea and fishing. I will die in Looe sat on the famous 'Banjo Pier'. Because I know the date, month and year of my death I am able to say that and plan it. It's a most privileged and comforting position to be in. To know when and therefore to be able to plan where and with whom is a real gift and advantage. Those I have shared this information with think I am in a terrible position but I just don't see it that way.

Once again, my glass is half full !

Stroke has meant my family has had a lot to put up with and they needed fun and laughter back into their lives so to have the promise of a Florida holiday with our dear and valued friends to look forward to was a huge and much needed boost for all of us. Friends can be instrumental in a recovery programme and I am sure that one thing which helped my recovery was the regular contacts with the friends I have. John Matthews is a former work colleague and I enjoyed our regular meetings and discussions. We often share deep discussions about the world, who is in it and how it operates! They were real bloke's chats. Most of it absolute bollocks but nevertheless we enjoyed it. John is insightful in what he says and most thought provoking. Our discussions on the meaning of life were always positive, vibrant, helpful and encouraging. We didn't solve anything though but we always seemed better for it afterwards.

> Knowledge Nugget – understand that whilst your life has changed dramatically friends are, generally, trying to maintain the normality of their everyday life. Some don't handle change very well.

My relationship with my wife was the area under most threat. I realise that she probably felt that her protector and strong reliable man was now broken and vulnerable and certainly not the reliable protector and provider he once was. I'm sure she was the most fortunate of the two of us because it is far easier to maintain the home equilibrium than it is to battle the effects of stroke. Nevertheless, we're a team and together we have to battle onwards and upwards for our family unit. Unfortunately some of our more usual family activities were hindered by the effects of the stroke. A trip to the cinema became a nightmare rather than a joy when I was still in a wheelchair such was the difficulty of transferring from one seat to another. A shopping trip was a virtual non starter on the basis that wheel chair access seems not to have been a consideration at the design stage of many buildings. It's sad to think that the world has not thought very deeply about the needs of disabled people for them to go about their everyday lives. Such was a shaming realisation for me because I was once a guilty party in that inconsiderate world.

Chapter Three

Initial 'Care'

A number of checks were carried out immediately as I was admitted to hospital to determine the extent of my problem. Not only did I have paralysis of the left side including a droopy face, my speech was slurred and my sight was affected with considerably impaired peripheral vision to the point of near blindness. Had a clot developed as a result of the operation and if it had how had it travelled to my brain? I still think the blood thinning medicine that was administered to me as I lay recovering from a hip resurfacing operation should have been prescribed to continue thereafter at home. It wasn't. A clot formed but the reason for it is still a mystery as highlighted in a letter from my DRI hospital neurological consultant, Dr. Nicola Brain (yes, Brain! That really is her name!) who, on 6 September 2006 wrote to the Department of Clinical Sciences at the University of Bristol stating:

'I have recently had under my care a 42 year old gentleman who underwent a right Birmingham hip resurfacing replacement in December 2005. Two weeks following this procedure he developed an acute stroke. We have not found any relevant risk factors.

Andrew Shaw

Obviously I am aware that stroke can occur after any operative procedure. However I would be very interested to know whether you have come across any other associations between this procedure and stroke, particularly in younger patients'.

As investigations continued soon after the stroke it was thought that I might have a hole in my heart providing a route for the clot to get to my brain rather than it travelling into the lungs and causing almost certain instant death. The medical view was that had a clot gone into my lungs then death was the most likely outcome. Whatever next? Earlier in the evening of the 29th everything was going along as normal and in no time I am another stroke statistic and being checked for a possible hole in my heart. At least it's still beating. That's a bonus. One thing that struck me was the thought of 'How can this be?' and Why me?'

I suppose the answers are quite simple really as I look back now. Firstly, it would appear that anything can happen at any time whether it be a sudden health problem, a stroke (when are you going to have a stroke? - tomorrow, next week, next year or in a minute?) or an accident and secondly, 'Why not me?' Things happen to someone all of the time and sometimes to you and me. This time it was me. It has always puzzled me that smokers are shocked when they get lung cancer or develop some other smoking related disease or illness including stroke. Smokers are inviting a stroke into their lives. They'll be sorry if they survive! I lived cleanly, ate cleanly, exercised, so to my mind, as I've told you previously I didn't invite the stroke along, it just happened. 'Shit happens!' and this

Weather the Storm

situation is really shitty! I suppose my experience is grist to the mill for those who argue a healthy lifestyle offers no guarantees of a long and healthy life and they'd probably be right based on my experience even though I'd argue, statistically, they're wrong. I was a sportsman - both a footballer (coach and player) and a vigorous exerciser, making daily visits to the gym (in years gone by I achieved a creditable 5th place finish at the Mr. Britain body building championships at London's Wembley Arena. My eating regime was disciplined and rigorous comprising over a ten year period, fish, fruit, baked potatoes, vegetables, boiled rice and water. I had a post- op stroke rather than a post – unhealthy life stroke. The stroke I experienced was not the accumulation of self inflicted risk factors such as smoking, drinking, poor diet, inactivity or anything else. Had I brought it on myself I expect I would be able to add guilt and regret to the burden. Nevertheless, my clean living has made it harder for me to accept what had happened whilst on the positive side my physical fitness has probably helped me recover quicker than otherwise.

> Knowledge Nugget - Our grasp on normality is, it would appear, very fragile and only a second from changing at any time. Live for today or for tomorrow? I suggest we live, as though there will be a tomorrow. I'm doing that right now.

I have no regrets. My hip was very troublesome and painful and caused me to walk with a pronounced limp. It needed corrective surgery(or should I have tried physiotherapy before the knife?) and when my surgeon visited me, as I lay stricken with the effects of stroke I told him 'Don't worry about this, I'm glad we did it'. I know he was as upset with what had happened as I was and I didn't want a man who had helped me so much to feel saddened in any way. He got a wobbly bottom lip at my bedside. I'm unlucky to be have added to the world's stroke statistics as is my hip surgeon to be burdened by what has happened. As far as I'm concerned we can both look back without regret.

> Knowledge nugget- what has happened has happened. There's no turning the clock back in this life. It's understandable to be saddened and angry but try to look ahead and make the best of what you have even though it's not always easy. Play the cards you have been dealt and try to make a winning hand. The future exists only in our hopes and expectations. Whilst ever your heart is beating you can carve out some sort of future nevertheless.

After part of a night in the Derbyshire Royal Infirmary's Medical Assessment Unit I was transferred to Nottingham's Queens Medical Centre (QMC). Two things occurred to me. First, I didn't even feel ill. Second, If I'm going to check out of this life then let's do it in Nottingham, my spiritual home and the home of East Midlands football rather than Derby. Football really is that important to me! When I briefly awoke days later in the dead of the night I was disorientated and desperate to pass urine. Unfortunately I was in the 'two minutes yet never' hospital as I came to discover. My experience of the QMC is that when politely asking for something, in this instance a urine bottle, the response was always a dismissive 'just give me two minutes' yet the responder never returned. Such was my desperation that as I recall it I somehow slid feet first out of bed, toes into the floor with my chest against the edge of the bed giving me a position to urinate directly onto the floor. I must have been desperate! How I managed to manoeuvre out of bed remains a mystery. Months later into my hospital stay I knew I couldn't repeat the feat which meant some wet beds and humiliation. However, in my experience of the NHS (with the exception of the stroke unit at the DRI) allowing a patient to sleep on a layer of warm piss and having to change the bedding later is preferable to providing a receptacle to piss in! What a disgrace, shambles and utter humiliation.

Stroke 4 Andy Shaw 2

The situation got so bad that when my parents witnessed the apparent disinterest of certain nurses and the two minutes yet never principle in practice at the QMC they were forced to take my care into their own hands even though I was technically an NHS victim - otherwise known as a patient. My parents were so upset, shocked and disgusted at my plight and could clearly see the distress the apathetic care was causing that my mother offered to stay overnight to be there for me. Of course she received the typical British politically risk averse answer 'We can't allow that. It's health and safety you know'. The outcome was that myself and other, far older, ward incumbents occasionally in the middle of the night wet the bed and suffered the humiliation that accompanies such. On one occasion in the middle of the night I couldn't summon a nurse to take a break from the gossip at the reception desk so I had no option but to urinate in bed and then try to position myself as far away from the dampness as I could. I recall a nurse greeting me in the morning with a cheery ' Good morning Andy, how did you sleep?' I responded caustically with a less than cheery ' Lying down in piss, what about you?' She said in reply ' Oh I see someone has woken up a little bit grumpy this morning'.'Grumpy?' I said 'Sleeping in piss isn't exactly my idea of starting the day off right!'

Stroke 4 Andy Shaw 2

I really don't think my words registered even though I'm sure she heard them. I found it laughable that much later in my hospitalisation the bedside bars were raised even though I couldn't have fallen out anyway. To get even close to the edge of the bed would have required some co-ordinated and controlled voluntary movement of my body but that seemed to be beyond me. To my mind raising the bars was unnecessary and time consuming and I was sorry that time could be found to do something that didn't need doing rather for something that did. I realise that it is something of a taboo to criticise anything or anyone connected with the nursing profession as the stereotypical view of a nurse is of a caring, hard working, underpaid, compassionate Nightingale - like figure. Many of them are like that but, in my experience, not all of them. Certainly some on Ward 10 of the QMC during my stay left a lot to be desired. I never asked for much, I was polite and undemanding. Unfortunately the stroke meant I was completely dependent on other human beings as I was trapped not by bed bars but by a dysfunctional body.

Stroke 5 Andy Shaw 2

Concern and fear swept over me in incessant waves. 'Will I ever stand up and walk again?' I wondered and asked the doctors who without exception replied 'It's too early to tell'. I felt both worried and ashamed.

I was worrying about me but what about my family? How were they? At least they were at home and well and that was a position in which I longed to be.

> Knowledge nugget-Sometimes it's forgivable to think of yourself first when stricken by ill health. Put your energy into recovery- you'll need it because you have a real battle ahead against stroke. Stroke comes with a sentence of frustration without tariff. Who knows when the frustration will subside or end?

The QMC felt more to me like a Victorian sanatorium than a hospital and I disliked it there intensely. I wasn't receiving much in the way of rehabilitative care in the form of physiotherapy and I felt that I was simply whiling away the time when I was so keen to get on the road to recovery. I felt abandoned by my country and its health care system. To some I'm only a patient but I'm a son, brother, friend, husband and Daddy. To the healthcare system I'm nothing but to my loved ones I'm everything.

In the daytime I found it easy to pass the time with regular visitors and my habit of people watching as I saw staff and other patient's visitors come and go. It was as easy to pass time than urine in the QMC. The difference being that time was just disappearing into nowhere whereas the urine was disappearing into my mattress whilst the nurses were passing time chatting . There were only five fellows, including me, on the ward. To my right was a young man who had lost his speech whilst the bed to my left was vacant until a young black gentleman named Chris took residence. Chris was a thoroughly likeable fellow but seemed a little disturbed mentally. I made my diagnosis based only on his regular threatening rants directed at whoever was in sight although not necessarily in earshot. Chris, it became apparent, was also suffering from severe epilepsy and I felt sorry for him particularly because he, like me, seemed to be receiving little in the way of care and attention. Chris also caused me to have concern for my own safety as he regularly pulled out his intravenous drip and swung it around causing droplets of blood to fly through the air and become spattered upon the walls, beds, furniture or other items and people nearby. I was concerned that a nurse, I, or another patient may sustain a needle stick injury. Worse was to come though as one night into the early hours of the morning Chris awoke the ward incumbents by shouting and thrashing about violently. He then hurled himself onto the bed opposite occupied by seventy-five years old Sid Hook. It was a frightening experience for all on the ward including myself and, I expect, particularly for Sid. I watched the events unfold with increasing concern as I knew I was unable to move, whether to get out of the way or defend myself. As usual the staff were conspicuous by their absence. I felt so vulnerable because Chris was not the sort of man who could be calmed by negotiation and soothing

Weather the Storm

words. More accurately he'd fucking lost it big time! Had I not been suffering the effects of stroke and been my previously fit and well self I would have been comfortable in dealing with whatever situation came my way. As it was I could not move. My left side was paralysed and my right leg was still immobilised due to the new hip. The only thing in my armoury was an operational right arm which in my body building days was my 18 inch 'gun'. I didn't have to fire it as the situation was eventually, after about twenty minutes, brought under control when a nurse heard the commotion, bothered to investigate and then called hospital security. Moments later two burly uniformed men wrestled Chris to the ground whilst the accompanying nurse administered a sedative and the situation was under control.

The following morning Chris was nowhere to be seen but the events of the evening were the subject of much discussion. Many were critical of Chris whereas I felt sure that he wasn't to blame. His condition was the cause and I always think 'that could be any one of us'. Chris probably wouldn't have known what he'd been involved in, the poor man.

Out of many situations comes humour and laughter. The 'attack' on Sid Hook gave us much to laugh about thereafter. It turned out that Sid is a relative of Henry Hook. The same Henry Hook who won the Victoria Cross as a result of his bravery at the battle of Rourkes Drift as depicted in the movie 'Zulu'.

Sid was quick to develop the story of his own personal battle telling anyone who would care to listen and even those who would not that he now knew how 'my uncle Henry' must have felt all those years ago! Chris wasn't a

Zulu but as far as Sid was concerned he was black and therefore fitted into his developing story perfectly.

Sid said 'As the Zulu warrior came over the end of my bed I quickly reached for my rifle but could only find a 'piss bucket' (urine bottle) so I thought if I can't shoot the fucker I'll drown him in warm piss instead!'

Sid's imagination and ability to develop a funny story were wonderful and to be admired. He is a funny guy. To his credit he kept me laughing for the rest of my stay in the dreadfully depressing QMC. I've met up with Sid since and his view of the QMC mirrors my own.

I don't know what ever happened to Chris. I only hope that he is fit, well and prospering. I know that Sid is still telling how he managed to out do the legendary Henry Hook. Sid didn't receive the Victoria Cross but I presented him with a urine bottle. Empty and unused.

As for my condition I constantly asked medical staff what was to become of me. Understandably doctors and physiotherapists seem to have mastered the 'non committal' response. To me a response that is guarded is negative. But eventually I came to understand their apparent reluctance to say more. I hold the view that they really don't know much about individual outlook for each stroke-affected person. For my money stroke recovery depends so much on the extent of the damage to the brain and the individual's mind set and inner ability to battle. Of course some stroke brain damage is so extensive that recovery is beyond even the most determined and focussed mind. When I asked myself whether I could recover the answer was a resounding 'Yes' and I felt sure that I could do it despite the fact that I had suffered 'extensive cerebral infarction (brain cell death)'.

Stroke 6 Andy Shaw 2

> Knowledge Nugget - I have no doubt that a positive mental attitude is the absolute key to stroke recovery.

Looking back I am sure that I did not truly appreciate the seriousness of my situation. Stroke? It doesn't sound like much. It hardly arouses concern or paints concerning imagery like 'Heart attack or 'Cancer'. Over recent years the term 'stroke' has developed to 'brain attack' or 'brain assault'. Still, I feel that the label 'stroke' does not highlight the seriousness and effects of the condition. 'Partial brain death' is a weak description but that's what we're dealing with as an outcome. Perhaps I am fortunate that I did not truly appreciate the seriousness of my situation. Indeed, the only things that I did appreciate in the QMC were my regular visitors, Sid Hook's humour and a beautiful young female occupational therapist named Charlie Morton – an absolute beauty.

Sometimes it's hard to be positive and, try as I might, I found it difficult to always remain up beat due to my immobility and the dead weight hanging lifelessly from my left shoulder. It used to be called my left arm although it was to be called something else later in my recuperation. It hung like a dead rabbit and I wondered 'will it ever operate again and find its way to something I'd like to pick up?' I expect it so to do because I am unwilling to accept this sorry and depressing situation. My hospital visitors tell me 'It'll be ok and will come back' but deep down we know that we're all simply hoping for a positive outcome. Hope is all we had but at least we had that. It's typically British to offer crumbs of comfort for something to grab hold of but I needed more than scraps to live off 'It could have been worse' say some visitors, 'Your right side is okay and that's your dominant side and it's only temporary' 'They don't have to manage with only one arm' I think quietly to myself. The word temporary became commonplace particularly in my wife's vocabulary. I can only think that in her mind 'temporary' means 'not permanent but tariff unknown'. She remains a source of optimism, as do my dear Mum and Dad along with my children, son Tom and daughter Amy and brother Mike along with my caring friends. What would I do without them? I knew I had to stay up beat for them. My wife told me

'Andy, this has happened to us, not just you!'

It seemed harsh to me as she wasn't suffering the effects that I was but she was exactly right as she was suffering the effects albeit indirectly and to a much lesser degree.

> Knowledge Nugget - Try to appreciate that other people are badly affected by what has happened too. Family, friends, work colleagues and anyone else who cares for your well being.

When speaking to a friend he told me of a young man he knew who had fallen from his motorbike and damaged his spinal cord leaving him paralysed from the neck down. He said, 'Andy, when I speak to you I always ask if you have any improvement with the arm, but when I speak to him I can't ask the same question because there will be no improvement. He will never recover'. It brought me right into the real world and prompted me to count my blessings. Whilst ever there's hope there's a chance. I aim to take my chance.

Stroke 6 Andy Shaw 3

> Knowledge Nugget – take Solace in anything positive. It can be built upon to help achieve and maintain a positive mental attitude. Think about good things in your life that you intend to get back to. For me it was family, work and football - although I strongly suspect that being entirely realistic I might never play again to the same level (but only because of my recent inactivity and advancing years !) of course at forty something I didn't have many more years of running around left in me anyway. I still intend to try nevertheless. I can still talk so I can still coach young players albeit differently than previously which will be a new norm for me. I'd love to referee a youngster's football match in the future, which would require me to jog, quickly change direction and point with both hands and arms. I intend to do it and it will be Utopia when I do achieve that particular goal! That's 'when' not 'if' !

My love of football has given me many years of joy and hope in addition to many positive experiences upon which to draw. Football is my first love and in football parlance on 29 December 2005 I had fallen behind against stroke but it was very early days in the match Stroke versus Andy Shaw with the score standing at:

Stroke 6 Andy Shaw 3

Would I come back to win?

I recalled one of Nottingham Forest's ventures into European Football on 25 April 1979 needing to win in Cologne, Germany, with the odds stacked against them after a three all draw at the City Ground. I now found myself in a similar situation..........in trouble against very tough opposition and needing to battle my way back. All those years ago in Cologne Forest's Assistant Manager, the late Peter Taylor, supporting the late great and enigmatic Brian Clough, gave comment to local radio on Forest's prospects after a scoreless first half under much pressure. Taylor confidently stated 'We've weathered the storm, we'll take them now!' He was right and Forest won out in the end! It's what I'm going to do too and what prompted the title of this book

> Knowledge nugget!- draw upon all of your life experiences to fight the effects of ill health. In my mind experiences fall into to two areas – those you've had and those still to come. Utilise both to drive you on!

I've carried Peter Taylor's words with me each time I have faced a difficult challenge and knew that in my battle with stroke I had to first weather the storm before I could think about how to ensure victory in the end. I had to set my inner self on a complete recovery and in my mind 'complete recovery' comprises a number of goals including a fully functional body, a full and fulfilling family life, returning to my work, coaching young football players

Weather the Storm

once more and driving again. The optimum outcome for me may be many years away yet I look forward to the day when someone who doesn't know me expresses surprise that I have had a stroke. 'You can't tell' they will say and their words, I know, will be greeted with the same joy I felt when I welcomed my children into the world when present at their birth. I know because I've already visioned it.

After a month in the Queen's Medical Centre (QMC), which was the most depressing time of my life (it really is that bad!) I was experiencing a full range of emotions. I could weep uncontrollably at the least little thing, which shocked me because I'm just not like that. I could also become downright hateful for little or no apparent reason. It might have been that to simply get to the toilet I had to be wrapped in a canvass body sling to be hoisted up and then lowered over the toilet bowl. Such an operation did little for my dignity, self-esteem, confidence and mood. I may have been grieving for the loss of the Andy Shaw I once knew. I had lost all control of my life and I didn't like it. Unfortunately my wife seemed to take the brunt of my mood swings and anger adding credence to the view that you tend to lash out at those who are nearest and dearest. I am convinced my stay at the QMC did little to aid my long-term recovery. Many nurses seemed indifferent to my plight and my access to physiotherapy was extremely limited and certainly nowhere near to the amount that was needed to get me moving again – but in truth, what did I know? I was in a whole new world with absolutely no knowledge of how my new world operated.

I now feel positive that the sooner a stroke victim begins intense physiotherapy the better and all the literature I have read since seems to support that view. The problem I was facing was that I was the type of patient the medical profession does not want. I had been diagnosed but for my condition there is no medicinal treatment to improve my situation. I have to depend on physiotherapy and the passage of time and I am therefore of little interest to a doctor. I didn't need treatment for the classic stroke causal factors because I didn't have any of them. No high blood pressure, no raised cholesterol levels, no tar contaminated arteries from smoking. I didn't really need the attention of a doctor. I needed a physiotherapist.

> Knowledge nugget!- stroke recovery is enhanced by expediting access to expert physiotherapy. Physiotherapists expedite stroke recovery, not doctors.

My recovery was not to begin in earnest until I learned I was to be transferred back to the Derby Royal Infirmary (DRI). A Nottingham Forest Fan being transferred to Derby! Such irony. How bad could things get? In hindsight it was a good move for me since the DRI's Stroke Rehab Unit is, I was informed, recognised as one of England's best units for stroke victims to begin the long road to recovery. I can now, from personal experience, fully endorse that view. On the evening of Thursday 9 January I arrived at the DRI resplendent in my red Nottingham Forest home shirt. My wife said I was asking for trouble going to Derby dressed as such. However, there was method in my madness, as I knew I would be on the receiving end of much banter and would need to be on my mettle to respond quickly and effectively. It worked. I got lots of verbal 'stick' regarding my allegiance but responded with rapid fire. It kept me sharp! As I was wheeled out of the ambulance at the entrance to the DRI resplendent in my red Forest shirt, two young men spotted me and each fired a look in my direction which seemed to say 'I hope you die you Forest bastard!' Oh, the emotion and strength of feeling that English football rivalry creates. Magnificent stuff and I love it! 'Fuck off you jealous Derby bastards!' I'd sooner be a stroke victim in a Forest shirt than stroke free in a Derby shirt! Fuck Derby County – they're nothing compared to us!

> Knowledge nugget! Try to be mentally aware and bright. Test yourself

My Forest shirt played a big part in my efforts to recover. As the Supporters' chant goes to the tune of the children's nursery rhyme H-A-P-P-Y 'I'm Forest till I die, I'm Forest till I die I know I am I'm sure I am, I'm Forest till I die'. But I wished to live, and didn't intend to help stroke cement its third place as the third biggest killer in the Western world behind only heart attack and cancer.

> Knowledge nugget!- utilise the existing good things in your life to work for you in you battle against stroke

In the match of Stroke versus Andy Shaw now being played out at Derby it remained

Stroke 6 Andy Shaw 3.........

meaning I had to play hard. I knew I was in with a real chance when my physiotherapy began on my first full day at the DRI. Two physiotherapists assessed me having mechanically hoisted me out of bed on a standing hoist. I had progressed from the canvass hoist due to improving leg function. It just seemed to be coming back to life a little but still nowhere near like it used to be. The standing hoist is a battery-operated contraption fitted with a waist strap such that patients can be hoisted into a standing position if their situation allows. In the therapy room for my initial assessment Ann Madsen, a student of physiotherapy originating from Liverpool was excellent and, as I have come to expect from Liverpudlians over the years, she had a great sense of humour. Ann was working with the DRI's senior physiotherapist, Jan Jolly who I thank for putting hope back into my life during my darkest days. Jan is extremely skilled with the most magnificent manner and sense of humour, beautiful natural looks, blonde hair and a husky yet velvet soft voice. Jan was to work with me during my stay at Derby and with her on my team I felt confident of victory as she set about getting me moving again and back into the match. She really is that good.

I also met a magnificent lady, Tina Buchan, whom I labelled 'Mrs. Doubtfire' due to her Scottish accent having an uncanny resemblance to the aforementioned movie character. Tina is the life and soul of the DRI's Stroke Rehab unit with her glorious sense of fun and optimism. She could brighten up the darkest room and I looked forward to seeing her each day as she brought such a sense of joviality to the ward and to my life. She's a staunch Derby County supporter though but other than that she's great! On one occasion Tina, who has created strong links with Derby County and the DRI's stroke unit, asked if I wanted to go to a Derby match. I didn't have to think about it as I quickly and flippantly said, 'I'd sooner have another stroke thanks all the same!' My early days in the DRI gave me much hope about my recovery yet one vital thing was missing for me probably because of the sort of man that I am. After the physio's initial assessment to determine the extent of the effects of the stroke I would liked to have discussed their findings and their planned treatment program. Perhaps their initial view was that I would quietly accept what they professionally decided for me without discussion. I'm just not like that as I need to ask questions and to understand. It might be the norm (albeit an unacceptable norm) to make decisions without consultation for a meek ninety five year old stroke victim but not for me. I can't give it my all unless I understand quite what I'm doing, what I'm working towards and what the benefits will be. It's not sufficient to know that it's for my recovery. OK, but what do I need to do and why? It's my body and it tells me things that, in turn I can pass on to a doctor or physiotherapist. I was told we were to work on my core stability. 'Core stability?' I said, 'what is that, what does it do and how will it help me?' I needed answers in order to think things through and understand where I 'm going so I have the opportunity to figure out the route to victory. I didn't feel satisfied or have confidence in what I was doing until a friend, Richard Staley, visited me and fully explained the need for core stability training. When he told me that he had worked on his body core to ease a back and mobility problem and that it had been successful I could understand the principles and it became credible. At that point I had understanding and confidence in core stability training to help me and therefore I gave it my all. Looking back, I think the problem was that I hadn't understood that stroke had affected my trunk muscles and that they are vital in the mechanics of limb movement. NHS Physiotherapists have been both a source of help and great frustration. They need to understand that imparting knowledge to their patient in layman's terms might help to beget performance.

> Knowledge nugget for physiotherapists- ensure your patient understands the effects of stroke and the need for, and effects of, the physiotherapy you are to employ to achieve the desired result. Communicate!

I accept that I wasn't the easiest of patients because my progress seemed slow and all day long people hammered into me the need to be patient. What they didn't realise was that I was fresh in from a fast paced, results driven life and it's not so easy to just change a mindset, particularly one that had allowed me to be so successful in life. After much frustration and tears I began to make steady progress. However my frustration was always bubbling away underneath a positive surface and each day that passed that I didn't get on my feet just added to the frustration. Again I was reminded to be patient at all times. On one occasion when seated on a plastic shower chair in the one and only shower cubicle on the DRI stroke ward a nurse bellowed in with an instruction to 'get a move on' I couldn't resist the obvious retort ' Be patient – practice what you preach'! Nevertheless I worked hard on the exercises I had been recommended. Often, the morning ritual comprised a washing and dressing assessment, which was most valuable to me once I got home. It's not easy trying to put on clothes, especially socks and shirts, with just one arm and hand operating. Constantly I had occupational therapists (OT's) seated behind me telling me that I was leaning to one side whilst seated. I couldn't sense it myself and that's one of the effects of stroke. I was prompted and prodded in an attempt to get me to sit up straight and I felt it was criticism of the posture that had served me well throughout my life. I certainly didn't feel any different when seated and I quickly grew tired of their comments and touching. I was close to touching a few of them with a clenched fist right on the jaw on a few occasions! I didn't appreciate what they were trying to do for me but why would I? Stroke plays tricks on the mind/body relationship. I was suffering from 'left sided neglect' caused by the damaged part of my brain. One morning, when shaving with my useful right hand I emptied the water bowl and put away my razor even though the left side of my face was untouched. I hadn't noticed that the left side of my face was covered in shaving foam and unshaven. To the non stroke person this might seem incredible but it's very real and true. It's fucking weird and disconcerting. Strangely though I was only to aware of my inoperative left leg, foot and arm so there didn't seem to be too many advantages. Of course, on occasion, I played the situation to my benefit. After yet another shitty, cardboard dry hospital meal I pushed the rubbery vile green beans to the left side of my plate. A nurse said to me ' Did you not like your greens Andy?' to which I gave the obvious clever retort ' What greens? I didn't see any! I found that much easier than saying ' Those green beans were like fucking armoured cable!' It was not unusual for me to leave the left side of my shirt outside of my trousers whilst the right side was neatly tucked in. Left sided neglect is an incredible but very real phenomenon hence when being prodded by physios and occupational therapists I got so angry because I could not sense or understand what they were seeing right in front of them. To me I was symmetrical and fine but the impression they gave me was that I was some sort of fucking idiot. An idiot I am not ! My brain didn't recognise anything on the left of me. Once again the physiotherapists and occupational therapists were practicing in their little world and expecting everyone else to accept and understand without the prerequisite knowledge. Theirs is a specialist discipline that I didn't understand and they didn't bother to explain even the basics. I know my anger and frustration was apparent but still no one bothered to ascertain the root cause of it. To be fair, at the time I didn't always know why I was so angry myself. I presumed it was one of the stages of grief, and I was grieving for the loss of my pre stroke life. One thing that I latched on to straight away was that the world of the hospital physiotherapist is a 'Do as I say, not as I do' world. They were constantly badgering me to 'sit up straight' (I thought I was !) and, when it eventually became possible, to 'get up from the chair without the use of your arm'. I watched them intently and they didn't practice what they preached. As far as I was concerned their advice, if not even followed themselves, must be fucking worthless. I viewed it rather like me telling my children to use the controlled crossing when attempting to cross a busy road but not doing the same myself. If advice is worth imparting it's surely worth following oneself?

However, all the patients on the ward looked forward to the days when they received physiotherapy such was the skill of Jan and her colleagues. Unfortunately the therapy was not available everyday which, I suspect was due to lack of resources. Wednesday was named 'Group therapy day' but for me it was no more than a cop- out from what really needed to be done. Group therapy, in truth, was no more than a gathering of patients in the 'gymnasium' for a game of bowls, velcro darts and hoopla. I accept that therapy can take a number of forms and a social gathering with easy chat, understanding, listening ears and a forum to express oneself might conceivably constitute 'therapy'. I wanted *physio* therapy not a fucking chit chat or parlour games. My selfish priority was physical recovery rather than making friends with persons 45 years my senior despite their loveliness. I'll make friends when I'm fit and physically operational. Walking again and functionally using my left side was more important to me than scoring 180 at velcro bastard darts or knocking over a few wooden skittles. I'm single minded but willing to listen and negotiate but I knew I wanted to put all my time and available effort into becoming physically whole. I could image a future conversation where I might say to someone 'sorry I can't help you carry that but I'll take you on at velcro darts if you want'! I use the term Gymnasium guardedly as in truth it was little more than a wheelchair storage facility which staff called 'the gym'. When myself and other wheelchair bound patients were gathered in there any onlooker would have been forgiven for thinking they were seeing a re-enactment of an episode of 'Wacky Races.' I think I was one half of the grusome twosome and, sadly Penelope Pitstop was nowhere to be seen!

Group therapy day was, in my view, a waste of time. I really didn't understand, and still don't, how bowling a wooden ball at wooden skittles with my unaffected 'good' right hand whilst seated snugly in a wheelchair helped my physical recovery. Such was my frustration and building anger I threatened to throw the wooden ball through the window but was warned by a nurse that I 'would be in a lot of trouble' if I did so. My frustrated and angry response to that was to say 'Why don't you fuck off and do something worthwhile because I can't be in any more fucking trouble than I am already in'. I couldn't walk, or use my left arm, I felt constantly fatigued, was depressed and separated from my wife and children. As far as I was concerned I had trouble aplenty and anymore laid on to my shoulders would have been worth the devilish fun of breaking a window. To top it all I was then warned about overusing my right side. I was flabbergasted at the ridiculousness of it all and I eventually lost my temper telling anyone and everyone in earshot 'what a fucking waste of useful rehabilitation time group therapy was. Jan and I crossed swords which upset me greatly, such was my respect for her. Nevertheless, Group Therapy was subsequently abandoned to be replaced by a Group Exercise class working on core stability, which was a good outcome for, I believe, all. No additional staff resources were required. In fact less were needed and all participants believed they'd had more therapy rather than a game of indoor bowls or Velcro bastard darts. I believed I had made a positive impact for my fellow patients and had achieved a positive outcome by standing up for what I believed to be right, which I've always been prepared to do. In this instance I 'sat up' for what I believed in as standing was still beyond me but it wasn't too far away.

On 03 March, despite the trials and tribulations that went before and almost four months after an acute and extensive stroke I took my first steps, albeit awkward ones, even though young nurse and therapist, Ken Winfield, assisted me at my waist. Ken was another key player in my rehabilitation. He is a young man with huge compassion, understanding and willingness to help with a great repertoire in mood lifting quips and one-liners. If ever a young man has been completely suited to work in the care industry it is Ken. He was a good man to have around and some of his female colleagues would be well served to take on and apply some of Ken's attributes.

Anyway, back to the match I'm embroiled in and I'm euphoric because I'm walking! Such was my relief I wept uncontrollably.

Stroke 6 Andy Shaw 4.

My leg still felt heavy and my left foot seemed to be pointing toes down toward the floor (known as 'foot drop' in the stroke treatment world). Jan decided that a splint was required much to my chagrin. To me a splint signalled 'disability' and that was hard to take. I was so upset and I told Jan that I didn't want it. We discussed it and she quite correctly stuck to her medically informed opinion giving me a full explanation for her reasons. I understood and therefore acceded. I'm stubborn at times but I'm not a stubborn fool and so long as I understand and can question the logic behind the rationale I'm prepared to listen to anyone!

This life has a strange way of teaching us lessons that but for twists of fate or other intervention we might otherwise have missed. On a hospital trolley I was taken to the Orthotics department to be fitted with a splint. A skilled 'splint fitter' worked speedily and accurately then before wishing me well and dispatching me back to my ward told me he had suffered a stroke two years previously. I questioned him intently to learn of his experiences and coping mechanisms. I took much heart from this chance meeting that I had almost argued myself out of. Isn't life strange?

> Knowledge nugget!- Take heart from those who have experienced what you are now going through. Learn from them.

If the stroke resulted in any positives, one is that I met Jan. I hope she lives a long, healthy and happy life. And if there is any sense of fairness in life then she will be forever smiled upon. Of course, many people will testify to the 'fact' that life isn't fair. I don't feel I've been dealt the hand I deserved because of the stroke.

> Knowledge Nugget – sometimes life isn't fair so we have to make the best of what we have. Try to accept what has happened and then set to work upon your recovery.

I have become very mindful of how I refer to my experience of stroke and, as I have already told you, always term it 'the stroke' rather than 'my stroke' as many other stroke victims seem to. I was, and continue to be, irritated by anyone who went against this. I didn't want to have a stroke so I'm dammed if I'm going to take ownership of it and let it become mine as in 'my stroke'. As far as I'm concerned it will always be 'the stroke' which came into my life rather like an unwelcome visitor. I made that point clear to all when they asked the usual question 'When did you have 'your' stroke?'

> Knowledge Nugget – Stroke and its effects is your enemy – fight it all the way

It wasn't *my* stroke. I didn't want it so please don't term it as such.

Such was my desire to have a say in my treatment I think the staff at the DRI's excellent Stroke Rehabilitation Unit will remember me! Some with fondness and some without!

> Knowledge nugget!- have your say about your treatment but be guided by a skilled therapist

I will certainly remember them, some with extreme fondness like Jan Jolly, Sister Jayne Gill, Nurses Brian Neal, Kevin Limbert, Eric Smith and Chrissy Jollands. Kevin has worked with stroke patients for many years and intuitively knows what they are and are not ready for .In fact he was the one who agreed with me when I said I felt I was ready to stand up when others who I remember with less fondness tried to tell me my own mind and body. Stroke seems to run riot with moods and emotions and I found myself on such an emotional rollercoaster that I could not get off. The slightest thing set the coaster racing uncontrollably for a whole day. At times I was a cantankerous, hateful bastard but other than that I was alright!

> KNOWLEDGE NUGGET- To be emotional as a victim of stroke is both normal and acceptable - let it come out whether you're male or female. The outpouring of tears is not a negative reflection upon manliness! Stroke plays havoc with emotions. It's tears one minute and then settled again the next.

The men's bay of the SRU holds just eight beds, four each side with a narrow aisle separating the toe ends of each and my stay was as pleasurable as a hospital stay could be save for the morning ritual which included an early awakening from a medication induced slumber by some raucous staff at shift changeover time as though they might never see each other again and had little consideration for the sleeping incumbents of the ward. The only way they could have made more noise is if they had been carrying biscuit tins containing marbles! What a commotion! Any doubts about their consideration were well and truly dispelled when the bright fluorescent lights were switched on. To encounter such bright lights after hours of darkness I found I incredibly disconcerting and unsettling and it really affected my mood. It didn't have to be like that as it was possible to switch smaller night-light on first and, backed by the other incumbents of the ward , I politely protested to one of the two ward sisters. My motivation was to be awoken without the shock of glaring light whilst my fellow ward incumbents merely wanted

Weather the Storm

to awaken in their own time. I understood their desire as their weekend days were empty save for an exchange of conversation (for those who still had the power of speech and understanding). There was no physiotherapy on Saturdays or Sundays thus the days were long hence the desire to be awoken later. Breakfast wouldn't be spoiled – the Cornflakes could just sit in the box! On behalf of the fellows I took up the case with one of the ward Sisters who wasn't prepared to act. Patients seemed to be a burden to her rather than the subject and very essence of her occupation!

I explained the situation courteously and fully to her also offering the simple solution rather than to simply drop a problem into her lap. She dismissed my request of a 'sleep in' and a reduction of the shock- inducing bright lights out of hand without due consideration. She didn't even want to discuss it and such was her unwillingness to even acknowledge the issues of something worthy of discussion I began to think she was in the wrong job. Care? She just didn't seem to! Compassion? She showed me none.

The entire episode prompted my dear dad into poetic action, with a verse entitled 'The Boys'

The boys in ward 2a decided one night,
That waking too early just didn't seem right,
After all on a Sunday there was nothing to do,
Just boredom between meals and trips to the loo.

So getting together they worked out a plan,
and which was agreed on by every man,
They'd consult Sister[name] saying it would be fine,
If they could all sleep 'til a quarter to nine.

[name] ignored the request but the other staff in their
wisdom, not wanting a riot ,
From Andy, Jack, Roger, John, Glyn and Wyatt,
The staff said 'okay we'll do that and see how it works'
After all there's no therapy, no physical jerks,
No reason at all to be gotten out of bed,
To just sit in their chairs and wait to be fed
Though there's no thanks to [name] but there is to the staff
No boredom again say the boys as they laugh

> Knowledge Nugget for carers- A minor adjustment may make a significant difference to your patient's outlook, mood and mental well being thus improving recovery potential.

When I raised the lighting issue again, her excuse was that she had instructed the staff to begin our day with gentler lighting but they just weren't carrying out her instructions. With ineffective managers like that there is little wonder that the NHS is said to be struggling!

By contrast Sister Jayne Gill was magnificent. Not only is she a beautiful lady, who for me oozes class and womanly appeal, she has an uncanny knack of being able to say and do exactly the right thing at exactly the right time. She is one of life's special people and each time I saw her I imagined getting closer to her. One evening with my frustration at its peak due to boredom, inactivity and sharing a ward with five other fellows who were mostly in their eighties and nineties, Mrs Gill asked if I could help with a computer problem at the nurse's station. I was only too pleased to help with what turned out to be a relatively easy fix as we chatted away. She made me feel useful again, lifted my mood and took away my frustration in an instant just as it was beginning to get the better of me.

> Knowledge Nugget- it's good to talk and express how you feel to someone who understands and can help. The warmth and love of our fellow human beings should not be underestimated. Fellowship and care expedites emotional recovery.

The fellow in the next bed to me was comical and loud – I liked him but I know some considered him a little coarse and overpowering. Although his given name was Anthony Earp he insisted on being called Wyatt for obvious reasons! I did consider whether to ask to be called 'George Bernard' to go along with Anthony's Wyatt! I decided against it! Whilst I am able to look upon my hospital stay at the DRI as mainly very beneficial I found myself very irritated when staff complained about their lot, usually an impending night shift or a perceived unpleasant aspect of the job. The last thing I wanted to hear was some healthy and able-bodied person moaning about their work or the weather. I would have given almost anything to be contemplating a day's work or a walk outside into the cold and rain. Stroke has given me a unique insight into what life is really about. I'm not going to waste it.

> Knowledge nugget for carers- Don't moan about your lot to others who would dearly exchange places with you. Count you blessings!

One morning I challenged one particular nurse concerning her persistent moaning about having to make beds and suggested that all patients in the Stroke Unit would dearly exchange places with her as we couldn't climb out of bed let alone make one, her response was 'Oh dear we'll be getting the violins out for you next' indicating that I was merely feeling sorry for myself. I was offended, upset and enraged by the callous bitch. One day she may well understand my hurt if she has the misfortune of personally enduring this bastard affliction. I'm a pleasant man but I did think momentarily about strangling her. I suppose strangulation with one arm whilst lying flat would be quite difficult! I was prepared to give it a go though for that unfeeling witch. I'll spare her the shame and embarrassment of mentioning her by name and I don't hold a grudge as no good comes of holding on to such things and allowing them to fester. My efforts are on recovery rather than resentment.

During my stay in hospital it was decided that I was well enough to be wheeled out to watch my daughter play football for her team on a football field local to the DRI. The game was drawn but the result of the match was secondary to me at the time. I merely wanted to watch Amy play and play well but found myself at the centre of unwanted attention as parents of Amy's team mates wanted to chat to me and wish me well. Their kind comments and encouragement were appreciated. However, I felt so conscious of the fact that the last time they had seen me was as a proud yet concerned parent standing on the sidelines shouting encouragement to my daughter. However on this occasion I was sitting in a wheel chair with a blanket around me to keep me warm. Stroke seemed to have taken away my identity, dignity and way of life and caused me to be embarrassed and ashamed.

> Knowledge Nugget!- Accept people's attention with good grace as they genuinely wish you well. Work hard to recapture the life you once enjoyed.

Whilst I felt embarrassed about being in a wheelchair in front of people who previously knew me as an extremely active young chap I also sensed their embarrassment. Should they say anything to me? What could they say to me? The difficulty others have with the situation was highlighted when a friend, fellow football coach and fantastic man, John Adams, known with affection as 'Addo' said to me outright 'Andy, I don't know what to say to you mate. I'm bothered that whatever I say will be wrong'. I felt genuinely sorry for Addo and the difficult situation he was in. He's a great friend and a lovely, warm, caring man. I admire him greatly and, as always, appreciated his honesty. I really do believe that to have a friend stricken by a devastating problem must be hard for the healthy person. Lisa saw one of my friends when she was out shopping for groceries and she recalls the conversation going like:

Lisa: 'Oh hello (name). how are you

Andy's friend: 'I'm very well thanks but I've heard Andy's had a stroke. How is he'

Lisa: He's doing alright and he's battling on – you know what he's like ! You should call in to see him'

Andy's friend: Is he taking visitors ? What sort of state is he in? Can he talk? would he know it's me?'

Of course the effects of a stroke can be so different for each affected person. As Smits and Smits – Boone (1994: xv) point out 'stroke survivors [can] become paralyzed on one or two sides, and may suffer partial or complete blindness. If survivors can see, they may not be able to read .... [they] .... may also be disorientated and unable to remember their name .... '.

Perhaps my friend was frightened that he might be faced with a shell of the person he once knew. I think that his self preservation instinct and self defence mechanism was at work thus he had decided not to visit. After he saw Lisa I'm delighted to say that he came that afternoon and I assured him that I was cognitively sound if physically restricted. He said 'Are you having memory and reasoning problems.?' to which I replied 'Didn't you ask me that earlier?' we both laughed and he was at ease.

> Knowledge nugget- the person facing you in the wheelchair is still the same person and should be treated as such. If you're not sure what to say then be honest as Addo was with me. It will be appreciated.

> Knowledge nugget- Try to make people as comfortable around you as you can. I weakly joked about picking up further penalty points on my driving licence for speeding in the chair – anything to break the ice and put people at their ease and let them know they could still converse with me.

Weather the Storm

After the football I was returned to the DRI and my son, Tom, wheeled me to the hospital restaurant for a hot drink where I experienced for the first time the frustration of being ignored caused by having wheels for legs. As we moved toward the drinks machine the blanket over my legs began to fall away and drape onto the floor. A well meaning and considerate lady walked into our line of travel, looked over my head and into Tom's eyes and said 'His blanket is on the floor'. I wasn't sure whether to start dribbling out of the corner of my mouth and begin mumbling incoherently to satisfy her stereotype or to say 'err, hello my name's Andy and I've got wheels for legs temporarily. I understand English,can think for myself and wipe my own arse. This is my son and he's helping me to get a drink but I can hold the cup myself without spilling it and am capable of making a choice of drink. However, if you want to accompany us then you may. In fact, when I've chosen my drink you can then ask Tom 'Does he take sugar ? -If you really want to hurt me' As it happened Tom and I each had a drink and stopped to discuss the episode and then quickly moved on to talk about the football. What Tom experienced was as unpleasant for him as it was or me. As far as he was concerned Dad is the rock, totally reliable and still able to deliver the goods on any level. I was saddened and worried that the restaurant experience might have undermined his confidence in me but it was probably a useful learning experience for him as he moves toward manhood. The event had an immediate effect on me and left me feeling so very low and despondent that I was in need of an immediate injection of hope and positivity. It came in familiar guise through Sister Jayne Gill who welcomed me back onto the stroke Unit. Jayne immediately detected my mood and offered to listen should I want to talk. I accepted her offer and my mood lifted. Again, she understood completely and was able to offer exactly the right words at the right time. I had been outside for the first time since I had suffered the stroke and it was another step along the long, long recovery road and I am easing my way back into the game.

Stroke 6 Andy Shaw 5

Whilst it was decided that I was well enough to venture out to watch Amy, strangely the stroke has never made me feel unwell except for that mother of all headaches. I always felt healthy even though my body didn't operate effectively as previously. Perhaps that just added to my frustration. I felt in my head that I could walk but my legs simply wouldn't do it.

> Knowledge nugget:- Sometimes the mind writes out the cheques that the body just cannot cash in

It is odd to be lying in a hospital bed whilst feeling well. It just doesn't seem right. I felt fraudulent thinking that I might be taking the space of someone in greater need.

Adding to my frustration further was my dissatisfaction about the amount of physiotherapy I was receiving. Again I was on uncomfortable ground as my programme of physiotherapy was probably helping me more than any other thing yet it became my greatest bone of contention.

The therapy was fairly regular (usually every other day), Jan was magnificent and I really liked her company although I incurred her displeasure by referring to my lifeless left arm as a dead rabbit. She argued that by 'depersonalising' my arm I would hinder its improvement. To bring a level of light heartedness to the proceedings I asked Jan during my physiotherapy the following day if we could 'work on Snowy?' - the new name for my left arm. My children used to have a white rabbit called Snowy. It died and laid long and motionless much like my arm! Despite my Tom Foolery to try to lighten the therapy session which was one of the highlights of my day I felt as though I was doing something constructive even though I didn't feel I was getting the slightest improvement in movement and when discussing progress with my elderly ward incumbents it became clear that I was undergoing physiotherapy of a similar intensity and duration of fellows forty and fifty years my senior. I didn't expect special treatment particularly to the detriment of others but felt that my progress would have been greater if physiotherapy was more intense and for longer. It seemed to me that the care was geared towards the stereotypical stroke victim e.g. the elderly

> Knowledge nugget:- Stroke treatment in the UK and perhaps even the world is going to have to change as the stereotypical belief of the age of a stroke victim is challenged and broken. A change in treatment methodology is needed as the age demographic shifts.

I knew I could handle any treatment regime they could throw at me. When exercising with Ken I was asked

'Can you hold that tension in the muscle to the count of five?' I could hold it all day if necessary. By comparison to the stereotypical stroke victim I was young, fit and strong with energy to burn.

Thinking that improved movement is as a result of physiotherapy then my simple hypothesis could be shown as such:

If Physiotherapy = movement then 2 x Physiotherapy = double the movement

When I raised my hypothesis with the therapists it was dismissed out of hand and not even put to the test because, I suspect, 2 x physiotherapy would have resulted in resource implications for what seems to be our already stretched and mis-managed health service. No one was willing to debate with me and my hypothesis was rejected seemingly as the longings of a desperate man. They were at least half correct, as I was indeed desperate. I was austerely told that stroke recovery is a slow process and to be patient. I was unable to walk properly and had a useless left arm but was told to be patient. Would you sit quietly and allow such a position to continue without challenge? I was repeatedly told that stroke recovery is ' a slow, slow process' and I felt then, that they have something of a self-fulfilling prophecy going on. It's slow because everyone thinks it must be that way. It can be expedited, of that I had no doubt.

Oddly enough, much later in my rehabilitation I was invited to be a model at a physiotherapy course in Exeter – more of that later. My letter of invitation read

'Thank you for offering to be a model for our assessment and treatment sessions for the students on the above course.

This is a very important part of the course that allows the students to transfer their assessment skills into actual assessment and treatments of a client. **We hope that you will also benefit from this intensive burst of supervised skilled treatment'.**

The invite was months after my claim that more is better and that I might benefit from an intensive burst of therapy seemed to concur with my hypothesis.

When will I ever be operational again? My therapy had concentrated largely on getting me back onto my feet , at my insistence. I was faced with a most difficult choice – do I go for two operational arms or two operational legs. I wanted to walk again and, to me, that seemed, at the time, to be of paramount importance. I underestimated the effect of life with just one useful arm, which was the case when I eventually arrived home and it caused me much frustration and heartache.

Stroke 7 Andy Shaw 5

Things will always be 'as is' or as they are if challenge to existing beliefs is not allowed beyond the embryonic stage. Physiotherapy for stroke victims is a source of hope and mobility. Scarcity of resources in this discipline is unacceptable in this modern age with the increasing frequency of stroke in young people.

Nevertheless, I continued my attack on stroke by continuing application of effort towards my recovery. It's a battle of both mind and body but I look this challenger to my quality of life full in the face and quietly say to it 'you can continue to do your worst and I will continue to do my best and we'll see who wins'. I kept trying. I've always been a totally committed to any task I've taken on and recuperation from the effects of stroke has been my biggest ever battle . I knew after a few days in hospital (my first ever overnight hospital stay) that I faced a titanic struggle which, of course, must be met with titanic effort in return . And so it was.

After three months in the wonderful and helpful stroke unit in the Derbyshire Royal Infirmary following a month in the horrific QMC, the time for me to leave hospital was approaching and a few days prior a nurse approached me with the words:

'I need to talk to you about your discharge'

I feigned horror! ' Discharge ?' I replied, 'I've not noticed it, where's it coming from?' 'Is it a creamy yellow green colour?'

The joke was either lost on her or maybe just not appreciated. She looked at me with disgust whilst I laughed like a naughty schoolboy. The following day in the therapy room Jan informed I was to undertake the Berg's test. A test designed to determine stability and balance. Jan said I had scored well whilst I was completely devastated and disillusioned by the experience as I couldn't balance on one leg, bend to pick a towel off the floor and place my feet heel to toe. I remember Jan's poignant words 'look how far you've come'. The problem for me was that our starting points were so very different. Jan was measuring from the first day she saw me as an immobile shadow of my former self. I was measuring against a mobile football coach who some months previously prior to being struck by stroke had been overcoming severe hip pain to demonstrate to young players an angled run before ably side-footing a football firmly into the net. More than that I was thinking back to the time when I scored the winning goal for England against Spain in 1990 in front of a hostile Spanish crowd. (Okay, to be honest I have to admit that the match was during a vacation 'knock about' tournament whilst on holiday in Majorca) But, back to my conversation with Jan, for me it was a case of 'look how far I've gone' as opposed to Jan's view of how far I'd come. We were both correct. I was so shocked at the lack of co-ordination of my feet that previously were so quick and co-ordinated on the football pitch. I was reduced to tears once more although I had to brighten myself up quickly as I was due to be representing the stroke unit on a stall at the hospital entrance to sell raffle tickets in aid of the Stroke Rehab Unit. In no time I was laughing again as I was accompanied by 'Mrs. Doubtfire' who could make almost anyone feel bright and breezy. Mrs Doubtfire said that she had some tickets for the forthcoming match between Derby County and Leeds United and did I want to accompany her. I told her once again that I 'd sooner have another stroke than watch that shower of shite! My wife said she was so proud of me in that I was devastated by the results of my balance test but I was still prepared to lay that to one side in order to raise funds for the Stroke Unit. I really didn't see it that way. There was a job to be done that might mean an easier time for someone unfortunate enough to be incapacitated in the same way in the future. I felt rewarded that I had done 'my bit' for others. Some people were quite happy to wander by without giving our efforts a glance and up until my misfortune I was probably just the same. I wouldn't do that anymore so perhaps stroke has taught me something.

Andrew Shaw

> Knowledge nugget!-Stroke is becoming more prevalent so please try to help fundraise to give victims of this horrible affliction a better chance of recovery.If you've bought this book then well done to you. You've helped, as I'll always try to do my bit for any stroke rehabilitation unit. You might think it won't be you but it's going to be someone today and that someone might be you.

This book is my effort to do my bit. Hopefully I have penned a useful account and reference for others who suffer stroke, particularly relatively young people like me.

I had a jovial time collecting for the unit and was able to be juvenile which for a fat bloke in his forties is always fun. I put on a sad face whilst sitting in the wheel chair asking for a few quid. Alternatively I stood up and used the tried and tested flattery approach when picking out certain women(the ugly fuckers) and saying 'Excuse me my dear, I'm collecting for the Stroke Unit and I'm sure if your genorosity matches your beauty then you'll be prepaed to make a donation'. All the ugly birds virtually emptied thir purses into my bucket! Mrs Doubtfire said in her Scottish tone 'Och Andrew you're a wicked, wicked man'. Indeed I was but the job got done nevertheless. With more time and ugly women I'd have had enough for a whole new hospital wing! With the fiver left over Derby County could have bought two new players to improve their shit team !

CHAPTER FOUR

GOING HOME

On Friday March 10 2006 I was allowed out of hospital. I walked off the ward as I had set out to do although it was apparent that anything more than a few steps at a time was going to be beyond me for a while.

Stroke 7 Andy Shaw 6

The timing was ideal as Forest were playing away at Chesterfield the next day and I hoped to be there. Courtesy of my good friend, Jane Carnelly, Nottingham Forest's excellent and efficient club secretary I was provided with a wheelchair access ticket to watch the mighty reds crush Chesterfield 4 – 0. Happy days!

The previous day I had left the ward with the good wishes of the staff on DRI's excellent Stroke Rehabilitation unit. To say I walked is true but the style in which I 'walked' was a sobering reality check for me – I was a disabled person walking with a stick at a snail's pace and that was hard to accept. More accurately it was a hammer blow to my self-esteem and confidence. For the last thirty years and more I've been able to come and go to wherever I pleased, whenever I pleased at a quick pace. It had suddenly and unexpectedly reached an abrupt and painful pause.

> Knowledge nugget:- Stroke is a *pause* and a turn in life, if the initial brain insult is survived. It doesn't have to be an end !

As I glanced back at Jan who was watching her patient leave I threw down my stick in a stupid grand gesture and act of defiance. I wanted to be the man I once was and wasn't ready or prepared to be disabled. My wife gave me 'the look' which I have had many times and which says without the need for words 'I don't approve'. She was right because the stick I threw aggressively to the floor was the same stick that Jan had painstakingly cut to length for me and patiently taught me to use correctly to maintain my balance and posture. I never saw it like that at the time. Without the stick I was not well balanced and walked slowly with my head down. Bizarrely three things dawned on me. Firstly, that throwing my stick to the floor made me look a right twat. Secondly, that from now on I would be a lot slower and, thirdly, on the positive side, that I would probably never step in dog shit ever again! However, given the choice, I'd much sooner be fleet of foot once more and step in dog shit daily!

> Knowledge nugget! The contrast of pre and post stroke will come to the fore predominantly when you get home and try to do the things you once did. I found it both difficult and depressing. It made me desperately sad but I came through it. As time passed things seemed easier. My physical condition remained the same thus I suppose I became accustomed to my situation and eventually reached a point of acceptance – not such that my determination to recover was diluted – far from it. I did get through this most difficult phase of rehabilitation and so can you. It will be hard but it can be achieved.

I thought that once I had left hospital things would seem a lot better. For a start I'd be able to watch Sky's Soccer AM again on a Saturday morning with my boy Tom by my side. The promise of watching my favourite show now I was home again led me to believe things would be a whole lot better. However, I've been wrong many times so far through this sequence of events and in thinking normality might return once I was back home I was wrong again. Things were much harder despite the care given to me by my wife and children.

> Knowledge nugget:-Roles change when getting home and everyone has to be mindful of the stresses each are under. Roles and relationships are part of our identity so some parts of our identity are lost and others come along to replace them. You might not be the person you were but that's not necessarily a bad thing. I've slowly learned to adjust.

I had been every bit the modern husband and father. I worked hard and put in many hours to make provision for my family. My typical weekday comprised rising at around 0430 hours to drive the 60 miles to a gymnasium in the SAS Radisson hotel on Manchester Airport near my office in readiness for an early morning workout followed by a busy working day ending around 2030 hours. I'm not complaining. I loved it although with hindsight I realise that I was pushing myself to breaking point. My hard work and commitment though might, I now realise, actually have caused me to be the architect of my own downfall. Had I worked myself to the point of stroke? I remain in no doubt that the stroke is to closely related to the hip operation for them not to be connected. However, whatever the cause I am broken and relying on the input of skilled physiotherapists to get me moving again.

Immediately post stroke and being back at home I could no longer drive my children to their football training or join in with them. I was desperate so to do and I was at risk of my impatience becoming desperation. I couldn't get into or out of the bath no matter how hard I tried. I couldn't walk my dog, Renfro, or mow the lawn. These things still have to be done but my wife had taken on the roles I used to fulfil and enjoy. My wife had become my carer and whilst she was happy to help, I didn't find it easy to take on my new role as virtual homebound prisoner. More accurately I found it excruciatingly hard to go from self-sufficient to largely dependent. It's not that I didn't want my wife or children to help zip up my jacket, tie my shoelaces, carry my cup of tea, help me into the car or whatever else I could no longer do for myself. It's not that I don't like them doing it. The thing is that I can't do it for myself. It's not just frustrating, it's depressing as well. The simplest of tasks seemed to be beyond me. Putting a shirt on and tying shoelaces with only one hand is not easy and it is hugely frustrating.

My arrival home would, I thought, be beneficial to my state of mind and mood. In truth it really just highlighted my disabilities. I felt that I had, to some degree, become institutionalised and it was to be an effort to break out of the hospital routine.

> Knowledge nugget!- Don't expect to pick up just where you left off. Getting home after a lengthy hospital stay is lovely but it's also testing for all concerned. Give yourself time to re-adjust but in my experience things do slowly improve.

It was hard for me to realise that I was no longer the provider or protector that I once was. I underestimated the effect that my immobility, tiredness and subsequent frustration would have on my relationship with my wife. She was still my wife but her role had changed to carer and it had an effect upon us both. She reminded me, quite correctly that the stroke 'hasn't just happened to you Andy, it's happened to us!' how right she was. One morning when I was thoughtfully lamenting my situation she was moaning about the things she now had to do. Mow the lawn, drive the kids around etc. I used to do all those things and so I told her that she was now finding out what it was like to be me! I said 'I'd sooner be in your shoes than mine' but her response shocked me completely 'Would you really?' she slowly replied. I thought 'Yes I fucking well would' but it really made me stop to look at what was happening. I was thinking about myself without really having too much thought about everyone else's plight.

> Knowledge nugget!- Be mindful and considerate of the effects of stroke on those close to you.

As far as I was concerned I was the one who was suffering the most because I couldn't walk ably, couldn't use the left side of my body and couldn't work or go out to wherever I pleased. I felt trapped and had gone from having it all and being able to do it all to my current state of incapacitation. I was a bird without wings and the mental anguish was overtaking me and getting a real hold in my head in the form of depression. I felt that my wife was complaining about having to do the things that I used to do, would love to do now but simply couldn't anymore. It really grieved me more than I can express in words. In fact this was a time when I felt the effects of stroke were really getting the better of me and I was having real thoughts about whether I wanted to continue living the life I now had. How absolutely weak and pathetic and very unlike me.

Indeed McCrumb (1998:129) experienced similar feelings when asking the question: 'Better dead?' as I was beginning so to do. Stroke and its effects were getting on top of me and I needed something to arrest the fall into the abyss.

I felt that the stroke had robbed me of my independence, mobility, self confidence, future, and eventually I realised after much internal questioning and deep thought that unless I got my fucking head together that the bastard stroke was going to get the better of me. Fuck that ! There was a lot at stake in this battle and second place against the effects of a stroke constitutes a monumental defeat and I was having none of that. No fucking way !

Chapter Five

Inspiration

By sheer quirk of fate things got better for me and I received a massive injection of hope and encouragement. Via a mutual friend I was introduced to Chris Dent, who coincidentally used the same hair-dresser, as I did. Chris had a stroke in December 2003, a full two years before I had suffered the same misfortune. My first contact with Chris was by telephone when I introduced myself and enquired whether he would be willing to meet with me in the near future after I explained my situation. Thankfully he agreed and invited me to his home. I looked forward to our meeting like a child looks forward to Christmas and it came a few days later. Chris came to the door and invited me in. I negotiated his doorstep slowly by use of my walking stick. Upon settling down to chat I asked Chris and his compassionate and kind hearted wife, Sharon, if any questions were out of bounds. To my relief they were willing to talk openly about their experience of stroke. I asked many questions about Chris's recovery so that I could get a feel for what to expect as I fight to recover as Chris has done. Chris appeared very well, was walking and moving his arms seemingly perfectly. If you didn't know he'd had a stroke you would never have thought it. It was impossible to tell. Chris looks like any other man you might pass in the street. I was very encouraged and heartened by our discussion and by the look of the man. More accurately, I was inspired and hoped to meet him again soon, which I did a few weeks later when he came to my home. As he walked along my driveway and up the three steps to my house I watched him intently and he saw me doing so. I apologised for my apparent rudeness and thankfully Chris accepted my apology by saying 'No problem, Andy. I knew and understood what you were doing. You were using my movement, as a guide for what might be possible for you in the future weren't you?' He was absolutely right. He was providing me with inspiration and I needed it. Furthermore it is my intention in the future to do the same for someone, perhaps, I hope as yet unknown to me, that Chris did for me. I do hope I can help someone. I'm only ever a phone call or an e-mail away. Chris returned to me the hope that had been fast evaporating. He'll probably never realise the effect he had on my life. Simply massive.

Stroke 7 Andy Shaw 7.

I'm bright again thanks to the most understanding and compassionate Mr and Mrs Dent and the continuing support of my wonderful family. My question of 'better dead?'was answered with a resounding and hard hitting 'No, you're not! You have a lot of life remaining - live it!'

I had thought that to be out of this life was a possible escape from the despair consuming me but one that I felt would leave too much damage behind. What would my children think of me about how I'd just left them and become a quitter? They need my love and support both now and in the future and would be forever scarred if I threw the towel in. I've heard suicide described as running away from adversity and 'taking the easy option'. I never found it easy just contemplating it. I agonised over what to do for many hours and days and painted all manner of shocking consequences in my imagination. Laughably and ironically, the biggest hurdle I faced in achieving the outcome was finding a method to 'execute' it. Hanging was out because I couldn't rig up a noose with one hand and arm and my fucked up dysfunctional body wouldn't allow me to climb or mount a chair to get the height needed to dangle. I couldn't pass gas myself in the car as I couldn't bend to poke a hosepipe into the exhaust and hold it there until I pushed in the necessary retaining cloth. I couldn't run in front of a bus because I couldn't fucking run! An overdose? - perhaps but I might feel better after the first few pills but, alternatively, if I wake up my liver and kidneys might be bolloxed up as well. Drowning in the bath was out too because I couldn't get in to it. Fucking hell! Options are diminishing and desperation is growing. I know what to do! I'll get my head together and get on with things and see it through like a proper man. The irony of the situation was hysterical. I nearly died laughing! A brief conversation with a football colleague shook me out of my negativity when he expounded 'I'm sure there are thousands of people laid in cemerties who would love to swap places with you. Come on Andy, get your head sorted.' Another conversation, this time with my friend and soccer coach Gary Atkin, made me realise that my dark thoughts must be put behind me quickly.

When I told him I had seriously thought of suicide he said 'If you do that Andy, by the time your family finish crying you would have been walking normally again. You have to stick with it'. As it turned out, Gary had lost his mother when he was a teenager, which he said was a devastating event, and one he has never truly recovered from. I listened intently to him, accepted his rational point and knew that I had to fight on. He might well have saved my life and my family a whole lot of pain and heartache. That very evening my son Tom obviously detected how low and downbeat I was feeling. He shook me out of my low mood when he said 'Are you okay Dad? You know I would swap places with you if I could!' I was moved to tears and said 'I know you would Tom, thank you'. My thoughts of throwing the towel in were dispelled in an instant. I spent the remainder of the evening sitting quietly with Tom wondering how I could be having such selfish, defeatist thoughts which if carried into action would inflict such sorrow on my family and friends? My death would sentence my parents to pain and anguish for the rest of their days. How could I do that when I love them so much? , What would my children think of me? I imagined Tom with his son in years to come saying to him 'Tell me about your Dad, Dad'. If Tom was brutally honest he might say 'Oh I loved him but he was a quitter and he gave up as soon as he was faced by adversity' I realised my thoughts were selfish, weak, pathetic and very unlike the Andy Shaw that I and many other people know. In my defence I can only highlight the depression that many stroke suffers encounter. Such was my desperation and depression at the time even though I realised my plight was nowhere near as desperate as many other people in this world but that didn't make me feel any better. I've never subscribed to the view that other people's misfortune should act as a 'pick me up' although I wholeheartedly believe in counting one's blessings.

> Knowledge nugget! – Try to develop and maintain a positive outlook. If possible try not to give depression the chance to get hold of you because its grip is so strong. Talk to someone you feel you can open up to and who will listen. They might not be able to give you particular answers but an understanding listening ear can help considerably.

I realised I had to break out of this depressive cycle of desperation before it became too late. However, it's not so easy to just 'break out' of depression. I never truly appreciated how depression could affect a person and I certainly have more empathy with sufferers than I did previously simply because I now understand. In times past I've been guilty of thinking 'Oh, pull yourself together'. That is not helpful and doesn't work. At times such as this when feeling flat, depressed and down I tried to think about what I still wanted to achieve in life. I tried to prefix my thoughts with the positive words 'I look forward to the day when'. For example

I look forward to the day when I get my book published

I look forward to the day when I can run again

I look forward to the day when I return to work

I look forward to the day when my head doesn't feel cloudy, muggy and stroke affected

I look forward to the day when I miss the bus and have to walk instead!

I look forward to the day when I can briskly walk out side to bring the washing in because it has started to rain

I look forward to the day when I have 'work in the morning'

I look forward to the day when I can go to Florida and walk around the wonderful Sea World and the other visitor attractions.

I look forward to the day when I hold my grandchildren in my arms

I look forward to the day when I push a trolley around the supermarket

I look forward to the day when I have to mow the lawn

I look forward to the day when I can wash the pots in the sink

I look forward to the day when I have to do a quick blast round with the vacuum cleaner

I look forward to the day when I can manage a broadsheet newspaper

I look forward to the day when I can climb onto a fishing boat and enjoy a fishing trip in Looe , Cornwall

I look forward to the day when I can drive a manual gearbox car again

I look forward to the day when I have a mountain of ironing to tackle

And on and on

I also feel I still have much to do to help others who are similarly affected. For example, I want to talk to and help encourage others to recover, I want to hear of how this book has helped someone get on and stay on the recovery road.

Simply enough I just want to be around.

Another person who provided me with hope and inspiration was Harry Krampitz, a Canadian fellow who I met via the Shelley Rehabilitation Centre. Harry had a motor bike accident leaving him badly injured with his movement significantly affected. Harry had an accident whilst dirt biking at his brother's cottage. He broke his neck at the C3 level. Harry was negotiating a curve on a trail through the woods but travelling a little too fast. He went wide, ran into a small tree and fell, not violently, off the bike. Harry was knocked unconscious but when he awoke, with the bike on top of him, he was unable to move. When his brothers, in race pursuit, found him one stayed with to comfort him whilst the other went to call for help. Eventually the volunteer fire/rescue department came and they stabilised his neck with a brace, strapped him to a board and took him out of the woods in the back of a pick up truck. The rescue mission was lengthy and complicated comprising nearly two hours of careful driving over rough terrain to get out of the woods and to the local baseball field to a waiting helicopter which whisked him to hospital for immediate treatment in an attempt to reduce spinal cord swelling and eventually surgery at Sunnybrook hospital later the same night to relieve the pressure on his spinal cord. To me Harry looks in pretty good shape compared to how he described himself previously. It won't suprise you to know that Patty Shelley has been a player in his rehabilitation programme ! Harry helped me deal with the slowness of a long haul rehab program and for that I'll always be grateful. When Harry came over to England in June 2007 for treatment we met up and had a few days out together. We travelled to Chatsworth house – a stately home in Derbyshire near to where I live. Bearing in mind what Harry had been through I thought he looked to be doing really well though he gave me a huge boost when he said ' Hey you know Andy, I'd like to be walking like you someday'. I knew then I was making progress. I hope to travel to Canada in the future to meet Harry and his family.

Chapter Six

Back To Work

Believing that recovery would eventually come pushed my impatience into the background. I had no deadlines to achieve with regard to my mobility as I had returned to work and, by October 2006 had increased my working week, with the approval of my doctor, to four days per week.

Stroke 7 Andy Shaw 8

The one missing day was taken by rest because of post stroke fatigue or a physiotherapy session. Other than that one day I was confidently and competently fulfilling my role in the airline after almost 6 months out. Really, I felt I had done fantastically well, thanks to my family, my occupational therapist, my then physiotherapist, Rose and my unshakeable determination to return to work to play my part in the airline and my boss echoed that view. She had been kind enough to visit me in hospital and thus could see the progress I had made. My first day back in the office was 20 July 2006 almost seven months after the stroke. When I first exited the lift to enter the open plan 7th floor of the airline offices at Manchester Airport. I was embarrassed to be seen as I was walking with the aid of a stick, so incredibly slowly and imbalanced. I felt much, much older than my 42 years and was intensely uncomfortable with what I felt were looks of pity. I believe I was a popular figure at the airline so maybe the looks I drew were of care, compassion and admiration. I hope so, as I didn't and don't want to be an object of pity.

> Knowledge nugget! – Given the option of admiration or pity set out your recovery programme to draw admiration. To be pitied is not an attractive proposition. Admiration remains for ever so long as you stay positive and drive onwards and upwards. Pity doesn't last for long and whilst ever you are drawing pity you are not improving as you should. Pity won't help you move forward. It doesn't engender a positive mind set.

> Knowledge nugget! – I'm not recovering from a stroke, I'm teaching and inspiring my children. The end result will be the same ! They'll be better prepared for life and it's hurdles by seeing Dad battle adversity with courage and dignity

Unfortunately my efforts to battle back to work were to be in vain as the airline, beset with financial problems, decided to dispense with my services in October 2006. I wasn't shocked as I took the view that it was an easy decision to make. If anyone was a candidate to get off the pay roll then it must have been me, the newly disabled guy who's contributed nothing for the first part of 2006 and who puts his physiotherapy obligations ahead of the demands of the business. In fairness, I don't feel that my departure was anything other than the harsh realities of business yet hugely unfair. I have no complaints about how it was done. I'm not naïve about how big businesses operate. They don't care about the hardship faced by one of their employees. That I was trying hard to recover from the effects of stroke wouldn't even register on the Company Reichter scale. That they thought they could get through without me and I suppose to take my hefty salary and benefits off the bottom line would be the most important and appealing thing. I had performed well for the airline and had added to their wealth whilst I had worked for them but the corporate body has no conscience and no memory. I'm not Andy Shaw, Stroke Survivor and hard working company man. I'm staff number 11244 and I'm gone with the stroke of a pen.

Stroke 8 Andy Shaw 8

As my solicitor, Lianne Payne informed ' Andy, business needs and finances always seem to prevail over humanity' I agree with Lianne who went further when she brought my attention the words of Thurlow (1981:386) who asserted '[The] Corporation is the epitome of the 'bad man'. It has no soul to be damned, and no body to be kicked. It has a preoccupation with profit and when presented with alternative courses of action, the question it will ask itself is whether it will be better off or worse off financially for having followed a particular course of action'.

In my case I don't think that was a cut and dried certainty because in my first two years with the company I had saved them more money than it cost them to employ me and I have no doubt that when informing me of my redundancy the Managing Director, accompanied by the HR Director, had a hard time delivering the news. I felt incredibly hard done by. I had returned to the office far quicker than was expected and probably far quicker than was good for me.

> Knowledge nugget! – Remember the words offered by Bryson! - work is a rubber ball and will bounce back. Don't, as I did, put the corporation before your own immediate needs. In my experience it won't be appreciated. Put your health needs ahead of corporate demands.

Obviously my efforts to return to the office were neither recognised nor appreciated. I would have been better off to have stayed at home and let time pass whilst getting paid. With hindsight I feel that it would be a foolish company to confine me to the scrap heap if still off work following a stroke. My return gave them the opportunity to easily cast me aside. Silly me! but lesson well and truly learned.

Although I had asked if my company car could be exchanged from a manual gearbox to automatic my request fell on stony ground. The exchange would be too expensive I was told! The unspoken message to me was very clear; 'we're sorry you've had a stroke Andy. It's unfortunate but not our fault. You're on your fucking own mate so deal with it'. I resolved the car problem myself at great personal expense but it was worth it both to drive to the office and recover some of my lost independence. I needed an automatic car to recover my independence. I mistakenly believed that my employer might give me a helping hand. Instead I was kicked firmly in the bollocks! 'Tough shit Andy. It ain't our problem!'

By contrast my boss, John Gaunt, at the Notts County Football Club centre of Excellence told me to try to recover the best I could and that my position at the club was secure and when I was fit again I could start back to work as a coach. I was so thankful to John for the boost he gave me because essentially he said 'I rate you as a coach and a bloke and I care about you and want to do what I can to help you'. John is a decent man and I liked him a lot. He's a hard man, a decent man and he cares. It was a bitter blow for me, John and the others working at the Centre when it's closure was announced due to lack of cash. It didn't hurt me financially because I worked there for nothing. I did it to be involved due to my love of football.

The loss of my job and income from the airline was the second stroke affecting me within 12 months, albeit this time it was the stroke of a pen and, quite frankly, I wasn't at all upset. More accurately, I welcomed the news as I had the security of a six-month notice period and was spared the fatigue inducing daily return trip to Manchester. What worried me more was who might be willing to employ me now. My concern was that I might be seen as a liability rather than an asset due to my physical impairments although apart from the time when

I worked in a coal mine I've never been employed for my physical capabilities.

Nevertheless, I recalled Bryan Bryson's words:

'You will soon understand that work is a rubber ball. If you drop it, it will bounce back. But the other four balls - family, health, friends and spirit - are made of glass. If you drop one of these, they will be irrevocably scuffed, marked, nicked, damaged or even shattered. They will never be the same. You must understand that and strive for Balance in your life'.

At the time I felt that losing my employment was minor compared with having a stroke so I didn't let it worry me too much. My greatest concern was how it might affect my wife, Lisa, who had enough on her plate taking on her new 'do everything' role – the role that I used to occupy with relish and without complaint. When I broke the news to her she wept, asking 'Whatever next?' My reaction was to cuddle her and say what I genuinely believed 'Don't worry, all will be well in the end'. My greatest concern was whether I would be able to fund the private physiotherapy treatment that I was so desperate to pursue. Lisa said 'things can't possibly get any worse can they?' although I had a completely different view and mindset. My family is healthy, I'm healthy but, for the moment, disabled, I'm improving daily, we have a roof over our heads and lots to look forward to, and Nottingham Forest is having a good season! The world is rosy! I thought things could be a whole lot worse. We were so much more fortunate than many and I knew it. The stroke has enabled me to count my blessings and appreciate my good fortune now more than ever before. I've had an extraordinary insight into life as a physically slow, restricted and vulnerable person. When I go to a 'hole in the wall cash machine' now I always feel threatened and vulnerable as almost anyone could take my cash off me at will. It might be that the elderly and young ladies feel like that all of the time. I understand and feel for them now whereas before the stroke I was blind to such vulnerability. It's hard to understand vulnerability when one has never felt vulnerable oneself. As Harper Lee told us 'You never know how a man feels until you've been in his shoes' Having lost my employment my visits to an automatic cash machine would be fewer and I had some hard thinking to do. What should I do now? Was I to concentrate on my rehabilitation or try to secure alternative employment? Uppermost on my priority list after the welfare of my children was rehab but I wanted healing for the 'whole man' and working makes me feel whole by giving me a sense of accomplishment, pride and self esteem. I didn't realise how recent events had devastated and shocked me. I'd had a major operation, a stroke and then lost my job. Three shocks, three hammer blows. The loss of my job caused me to feel very bitter. The decision was taken by people who could, I feel, have stuck by me a while longer but weren't prepared to. They almost crushed the life out of me, with the help of a stroke, and did it for the sake of the balance sheet. I think I'm worth a bit more than that. Most family men have three main pillars in their life – family, work and their health. Two of my pillars had been knocked over but, thankfully, I still had my family with me – the most important pillar!

When considering the healing I needed I wanted to return to my previous life, or something close to it - full mobility and total limb use preferred. My options going forward now were limited and I took the advice of my good friend John Gilbertson who gave me some tough love and said 'Andy, don't spend time lamenting your situation, just build a fucking pillar!' John then helped me a great deal by offering me unpaid work at his consultancy business in the midlands. The arrangement suited me nicely, I was more interested in getting up with purpose each morning than wanting a financial arrangement. If John's good enough to help me then I'm good enough to do it for free !

After many months of job searching I eventually secured alternative employment at a manufacturing company in Burton Staffordshire near to where I live. The offer of the job helped in so many ways. My self respect returned almost in an instant and, thankfully, meant an end to my humiliating visits to the job centre where the staff spoke to me as though I were on the scrap heap and a drain on the rest of society. During my job centre visits I didn't take kindly to being asked if I could read and write. The answer to that would be obvious after a short conversation. Furthermore, I didn't appreciate being told, when I asked what date it was 'It's the first of December. You write that zero one, one, two, zero seven'.I thought' Thank you very much you condescending bastard, the gentleman in front of you is well educated including a Master of Science degree and is only here because his employer was too quick to pull the trigger after he had suffered a severe stroke so get fucked!'.

The new job looked promising enough although I had a minor hiccup at interview stage when they asked what I'd been doing since the stroke. I said 'I've been working for a safety consultancy on an unpaid basis to satisfy myself that I can still cut it in the corporate world' The interviewer said with a hint of disbelief in his voice ' Mr. Shaw, no one works for nothing !' to which I replied ' You do if you've experienced what I have' I received another look of disbelief but still managed to secure the job. It was an easy and quick drive from my home, I would be working in the discipline in which I excel and am comfortable and the money was decent if not what I had previously earned but I really didn't care at all about that. The key thing for me was to feel useful again.

> Knowledge nugget! – Stroke rips away the self esteem and confidence like a wall being flattened by a tank. Think about the things that can repair the damage and try to rebuild the wall brick by brick. Eventually the wall will reach the height it once was. More than that, you have the opportunity to build a better wall.

Unfortunately my return to the workplace was short lived at just four months when my new boss known by some in the business as 'Inspector Clouseau' or Gordon Fuckwit the clueless cunt, the most incompetent buffoon I ever had the misfortune to encounter, told me I was taking too much time out of the office for physiotherapy. I was flabbergasted ! It had been agreed at interview stage that I would be allowed time to continue my rehabilitation which amounted to no more than two hours per week. My anger, which was constantly bubbling underneath, came to the fore as I told the clueless cunt in no uncertain terms that if he thought I was going to put the needs of the business ahead of my own physical recovery he could fuck right off! As it turned out, his boss, one of the company directors got involved in an attempt to smooth the situation over. I apologised for my outburst, foul language and lack of professionalism which was duly accepted but I was, quite rightly, shown the door. I couldn't really have expected any other outcome and I didn't try to fight it even though I put my case forward clearly and concisely.

The director apologised for 'Clouseau's' mismanagement and said it was the policy of the company to support employee rehabilitation.

> Knowledge nugget! – A company policy is only as good as the people who carry it into action or not, as the case may be.

I felt very upset and undermined but proud of myself that I had recovered enough to stand up and fight for what I believed in. Had I have 'rolled over' and cut back on my physiotherapy needs I might never have forgiven myself but I left with my pride and self respect intact although I was once again without an income. I often think how I might have felt if I'd rolled over and acceded to his insensitive and selfish request to cut back on my physiotherapy. I'm sure that if in 5 years time if I was still in employment but still physically disabled I would hate myself even more than the useless insensitive shit head I had the misfortune of reporting into. He can go to fucking hell as far as I'm concerned and one day, if he ever has a stroke he might think he's arrived there. He might also think of me. I hope he does both !

> Knowledge nugget! — Of course self respect can't be spent at the grocery store but I'd sooner be without money than self respect.

As I continued my recovery through home visits from community physiotherapists Kevin Greaves and Lisa Sewell I received a call from a physiotherapist at a local NHS hospital inviting me to outpatient therapy. Kevin and Lisa both helped me as much as they could although, try as we might, my left arm was not as responsive as I wanted but I was not yet ready to give up thus my fight to achieve my recovery goals will go on so long as I have the input of a skilled and able physiotherapist. The local hospital had such a person who I shall call Rose. Rose has a no nonsense approach which I probably need as I have a tendency to fool around to try to lighten up the proceedings. I got the feeling Rose had no time for my Tom Foolery and I had no argument with that. My wife often says I need reigning in at times. I've a tendency to talk too much and to act the idiot like a stupid little boy. Rose worked diligently to try to get results against the goals and objectives we discussed and agreed. My only criticism, which I raised with her, was that our objectives setting did not follow the 'S-M-A-R-T' format of specific, measurable, achievable, realistic and timebound. Together, Rose and I set several objectives including being able to jog over five yards and to use my left hand and arm functionally at the dinner table. I longed to be able to sit in a restaurant and eat a steak as I had done in years gone by. Better still if I could jog to a restaurant before eating my meal! I was keen to put dates against the objectives as I had done with Jan in the DRI though now I have come to realise that aspects of stoke recovery are not like birthdays in that they arrive on a known date. I've learned to be patient. Nevertheless I wanted dates to focus upon in the hope that I might get some 'end' point in mind. To be fair, I now realise that it can't happen quite like that as stroke recovery is far from being an exact science. However, I did feel buoyed that Rose felt a jog and some functional arm movement were realistic goals to set.

I was also receiving Occupational Therapy at the same Derbyshire hospital from an Occupational therapist I will call Tracy. Tracy is , an extremely understanding and empathetic lady. I really liked her and felt comfortable chatting to her. My appointment times were 1.30 p.m each Tuesday but Tracy kindly agreed that I could arrive at 1.15 so that we could spend time chatting. I found our chats hugely therapeutic, helpful and encouraging. I looked forward to seeing her. She made it clear she was not a qualified counsellor and I knew that. I didn't want a counsellor; I wanted a friendly face, an understanding ear and a thoughtful responder. Tracy was all of those things in addition to being a good Occupational therapist or 'OT' as they are known. I was grateful for her help and for me she went above and beyond the call of duty with her willingness to listen and talk.

Understanding, compassion and flexibility was something I needed from the out patient physiotherapy department when after about nine months of treatment to disappointing effect I decided I wanted to pursue private physiotherapy at the Shelley Rehabilitation Centre in

Weather the Storm

Giltbrook, Nottinghamshire. I decided to pursue private therapy as I was feeling increasingly frustrated with the rate of my physical recovery and the repetitive treatment. I didn't find Rose to be a particularly 'hands-on' therapist though I never really considered it until I began treatment by Patty Shelley at the Shelley Rehabilitation clinic in Giltbrook, Nottinghmshire. I discovered Patty by chance. My mother happened upon a local sports physiotherapist, Helen Smith. Mum told Helen of my situation and subsequently Helen strongly recommended Patty Shelley as someone who might be able to help me. I immediately wanted to follow up the lead of hope given because I wasn't getting anywhere near the rate of progression I had hoped for with the NHS at the local hospital. I now recognise that what I wanted compared to what was possible was probably unrealistic given the resources I had at my disposal but my desire for a return to physical completeness had become a personal crusade and I had to explore every avenue to expedite my return to fitness and mobility. Patty Shelley came highly recommended not just as an extremely skilled neurological physiotherapist renowned for getting results, which is exactly what I had always hoped for, but as the best 'neuro physio ' in the world.

Rose said she understood my desire to explore all rehabilitation possibilities and admitted she would do the same in my position. She knew of Patty Shelley and that she was a world renowned therapist. More than that, Tracy, who also knew Patty, labelled her 'The woman with the magic hands' and gave her a glowing verbal reference. Tracy had previously undergone training with

Mrs Shelley, who is a world renowned specialist in Bobath treatment of stoke survivors. My first visit to Mrs Shelley on 02 November 2006 told me Patty was exactly what I needed, she wasn't just fresh from the classroom and likely to struggle to make improvements in me if the problems she encountered weren't covered in a recently read textbook. A stroke affected left side complicated with a right hip resurfacing is not in the stroke treatment textbook She is a freethinker, problem solver and specialist who can work beyond the boundaries of traditional beliefs and practices.

Rose, after consulting her immediate manager gave me her blessing to go ahead and access the private care of Patricia Shelley with an NHS political caveat that I couldn't continue with NHS physio as well as seeing another physiotherapist. I was told I had to choose. I was grateful of the honesty Rose displayed but, in truth, wasn't waiting for her approval. I'd made up my mind to do the right thing for me, not to appease the whims of the NHS. I hadn't realised that looking to private care, as an NHS patient was a 'no – no' due to hospital politics. However, I had no time or inclination to negotiate a political minefield. I was interested only in my recovery and placed more importance on my wellbeing than politics. I was told by Rose in no uncertain terms that NHS therapists could not converse and co-ordinate with a 'private therapist' as they termed it.

I had to try to access Mrs. Shelley's care as I didn't want any 'what ifs' to look back on in years to come but upon enquiring about how I might become a patient at the Shelley Rehabilitation Centre I discovered I needed a medical referral which hip surgeon Andrew Manktelow

Weather the Storm

was only too pleased to provide. He's such a caring and skilled professional. I am lucky to have made his acquaintance. When reading Kirk Douglas's account 'My stroke of Luck' he tells of an occurrence at the Seattle Special Olympics. It makes me think of Andrew Manktelow. Douglas (2002:193)informs: 'A story was told to me about the nine contestants, all physically or mentally disabled, assembled at the starting line for the hundred-yard dash. At the gun, they all started out, not exactly in a dash, but with a relish for running the race to the finish and winning. All, that is, except one little boy, who stumbled on the asphalt, tumbled over a couple of times, and began to cry. The other eight heard the boy cry. They slowed down and looked back. Then they all turned around and went back …. Every one of them. One girl with Down's syndrome bent down and kissed him and said, 'This will make it better'. Then all nine linked arms and walked together to the finish line ….'

My post stroke world hasn't been quite so sugary sweet as that but it's had its moments.

Andrew Manktelow is the type of person who would stop and go back.

The hip he operated on is now working perfectly and all would have been well had I not been affected by stroke but I was and I have to get through its effects.

> **Knowledge Nugget** Hard things are put in our way, not to stop us, but to call out our courage and strength.

Chapter Seven

Patty Shelley

Patty Shelley came highly recommended from people both inside and outside of the healthcare industry and having met or conversed with several of her patients it is clear she is warmly regarded and respected.

On 2 November 2006 my wife drove me to the Shelley Rehabilitation Centre for an 11 a.m. appointment with the renowned Mrs Shelley. Within a few moments of meeting Patty I knew we were going to get along and work well together. She reminded me of me! What I still didn't know was the thing most important to me – would Patty be able to make me physically whole again? My goals remained very much the same and immediately she gave me confidence in her ability when explaining how she intended to assess me to inform how I might be treated. Patty is, I think it's fair to say, something of a maverick in the field of neurological physiotherapy and I quickly detected her methods were far from conventional. Patty is to physiotherapy what Brian Clough was to football. She told me that she couldn't promise anything but she delivered results and such was obvious when speaking to fellow patients all of whom spoke about her in the most glowing terms. Of all the physios I spoke to about Patty everyone was in awe of her talent and talked about her in the most complimentary terms although I felt their comments were prinkled with a smattering of jealousy. I feel they were threatened by her capacity to get results, such is her brilliance, and whilst I was excited about the prospect of getting back to something near to my former physical self I am nobody's fool. I know that talk is cheap. Fulfilling claims is much harder than making them although Patty didn't make any promises. I truly felt Patty was the woman for me but only time would tell. In comparison to the other physios I had encountered Patty is on a different planet. Far and away better. After seeing Patty I felt hopeful for the future but, once more, I returned to the issue of patience. Here we go again!

Importantly, I left Patty's practice with my hope of recovery still intact and for that I was grateful. I had been nervous that her expertise during the assessment might result in bad news about the likelihood of recovery. It was quite the contrary as it turned out. Patty informed me that I had 'lots of recovery potential'.

Stroke 8 Andy Shaw 9

I was delighted and so impressed by her that I immediately asked for another appointment, which seemed to make her uncomfortable. Patty quickly made it clear to me that I was the one to determine the frequency of treatments and that I would be the one who determined when I should be discharged. She appeared to me to be reluctant to drive the programme of therapy perhaps,

Weather the Storm

I suspect, due to the cost. I believe I am correct in my view that Patty is not in the physiotherapy business to make money but to help people. Indeed, I'm certain of that. She is a 'people person' and has a natural gift to handle and heal the human body. Moreover Patty is, like Andrew Manktelow, the type of person who, if involved in the Seattle Special Olympics, would go back and help everyone else over the finish line.

Unfortunately, things turned sour between me and the NHS physios. I asked the local physiotherapy department if they would be willing to speak with Mrs Shelley to ensure their methods were complimentary as opposed to negating each other. I wanted Rose to come with me to the Shelley Rehab Centre but her NHS bosses, she told me, considered that to be completely out of the question. My simplistic view was that cooperation and co-ordination between therapists could only be good and I felt Rose could learn much from Patty who, after all, teaches the world respected BoBath approach for neurological recovery including cerebal palsy and stroke. Despite the political posturing of the local NHS Hospital Physiotherapy Department I put a stop to their unfeeling, inhuman politicking by telling them I no longer required their physiotherapy '*services*' and they could consider themselves discharged from my treatment plans. I had to step away from their political games as I could feel depression and ill health descending upon me. Mental well being is critical to overall recovery thus I decided to vigorously follow my instincts, which told me to go for all out effort to recover my physical well being , thus sticking with the wonderful, naturally talented Mrs Shelley. Such was the turning point on my recovery road and put me in the fast lane where I wanted to be. I told Patty what I'd done and she, quite rightly, distanced herself from my decision making. Nothing she said influenced my decision to steer clear of the politics of the NHS. I was influenced by her knowledge of anatomy and her wonderful healing hands.

I really feel that Patty works hard for her money and puts everything into what she does. At the local hospital's physiotherapy department I got the distinct impression that the primary focus was on the wall clock to see if it was 'home time' safe in the knowledge that, outputs are not critical to earning capacity and 'the money's in the tin'. I've seen that before when I spent thirteen years working as a coal miner in the National Coal Board which then became British Coal. I can smell lethargy a mile off and I can't accept it at any price whether I'm digging for coal, trying to win a football match or repairing my body!

> Knowledge Nugget – Stroke recovery is hard work for everyone. Everything has to be right to maximise the likelihood of recovery and all the players in the game have to be giving their all and pulling in the same direction. There's no room for politics, negativity and slackers. As with any team, those who aren't doing their bit have to go. Get rid and quick !

Chapter Eight

The Healthcare Industry

Since the stroke I have spoken to many people affected by ill health including stroke and other serious health issues. Their experiences, along with my own, lead me to the unshakable belief that not all in the health care industry actually care at all. Within the collective term of 'the industry' I include insurance companies, hospital staff, doctors and therapists.

I experienced an unfortunate occurrence with my health insurance company, Medisure, who provided cover for me as part of my benefits package as a Director of the airline. When Medisure was called to advise that I'd suffered a stroke their reaction was to say that if I was in an NHS hospital then it wasn't for them to put me elsewhere. Months later when I'd been discharged from hospital I called Medisure to ask if they could support me in accessing private physiotherapy I was dismissed without discussion with the statement 'we can't fund something where there is no guarantee that your condition will improve'. They couldn't possibly make such a statement without asking for an informed opinion. I wasn't shocked but I was disappointed.

> Knowledge Nugget – It seems to me that some healthcare providers excel at taking premiums and then becoming distant when their help is needed that might eat into their profits! I don't trust the fuckers!

Like many of the people I have spoken with during my recovery period I have no faith in medical insurance companies. Medisure was clearly more interested in their balance sheet than me and my recovery. I'm not naïve. I know they're in business only to make a profit or they won't be in business for long. Unfortunately profit seems to take precedence over the well being of people. As far as I was concerned Medisure had received their premium but weren't willing to help me in my quest for private physiotherapy. I was disgusted, if not shocked, that my needs were discarded without consideration or a second thought. What I wonder about most is whether these people can actually sleep at night! Medisure's opinion was trotted out without thought or the necessary information to take such a stance. Indeed Patty Shelley's view was that I had 'lots of recovery potential'.

Medisure weren't alone in treating me with disdain. Nottingham's private Park Hospital where I underwent my hip operation took joint 1st in the 'lack of care and compassion' stakes. By contrast hip surgeon Andrew Manktelow has been terrific throughout. During a pre-operation assessment I was issued with a raised lavatory seat, a pair of surgical stockings and a handled tool designed to allow me to pick articles from the floor without necessitating bending. At no time was I advised that the items were to be paid for. They simply informed me that they were necessary so as not to put stress onto the new joint and wound. I presumed, wrongly, that they were a complimentary part of the recovery process. For a complete newcomer to surgery I don't think that's unreasonable. I learned differently when, about a year later, I received a letter demanding payment for the aforementioned items which was soon followed by a stern telephone call ordering me to pay quickly or face the consequences. My response was obvious under the circumstances when informing ' I had a stroke following an operation at your hospital and the first contact that is made with me is one with a threatening tone demanding money rather than an enquiry about my wellbeing'. If at the pre- op assessment the need for payment was made clear I would have paid without question. They should have been honest, open and straight rather than running an underhanded grubby little money making sting. Furthermore, a short time after coming out of hospital I began to receive letters and telephone calls from the Park Hospital. Such contact was the first contact I'd had from the Park post stroke other than seeing Mr. Manktelow for a follow up on my new hip. Mr Manktelow was most concerned about my situation. Simply, he has compassion and he cares.

The letters and calls from the Park kept coming with a slight change of reason for wanting money – this time, apparently, I owed an excess on my healthcare policy which, since my redundancy, was no longer in force.

Andrew Shaw

On 26 January 2007 I received a letter from the Credit Control Department of the Park Hospital as follows:

Dear Mr Shaw,

According to our records, and despite reminders sent to you, the balance on the above invoices of £126.00 is still outstanding, due to the excess on your policy.

The amount is now overdue, and we must ask you to send your remittance in the next few days, to avoid further action.

If you wish to pay over the telephone by debit/credit card, please contact our cashier on [telephone number].

> *[Name]*
> *Credit Control*
> *The Park Hospital*
> *Sherwood Lodge Drive*
> *Burntstump Country Park*
> *ArnoldNottinghamNG5 8RX*

I was most disturbed and upset to receive such a letter particularly with the threat of further action.

At no time did they ever write or call to say 'How are you Andy?'

I replied with venom and emotion:

29 January 2007

Dear Ms. [name],

'Thank you' for letter of 26 January 2007 demanding payment of £126.00 which you inform to be due to an excess on my healthcare policy.

Please allow me to explain my current situation.

On 13 December 2005 I was admitted to the Park Hospital under the expert care of Mr. Andrew Manktelow for a Birmingham hip resurfacing operation.

Whilst the operation went well and the hip seems now to have made an excellent acute recovery I suffered a severe stroke just 16 days later due to a postoperative blood clot.

I can assure you that it is not to be too dramatic or sensational to say that the stroke has shattered my life and that of my young family. As an additional complication of the effects of the stroke I have since lost my employment and income. It has not ruined my life completely. I won't allow that to happen although I have in recent months been thrust into the dark world of suicidal depression.

I am sure you will appreciate my disappointment that the only contact from your hospital is of a type demanding money. It says much that you demand money before enquiring about my welfare. Many people die from stroke so I have much to be thankful for although most of the time I find it difficult to see the situation with any positivity.

From your point of view I suppose my death would be seen as a loss of £126.00 rather than a waste of life and a grieving family.

Stroke is a most horrendous affliction and in excess of 12 months post event I am still suffering terribly from its effects including paralysis of the left side of my body which, of course, is manifested in a difficulty walking, an inability to move my left arm and a functionally useless left hand.

I suppose, [name], that the explanation of my current circumstances has not answered your final and persistent question of 'what about the money?' It wasn't intended to!

The best I can do at the moment, [name], is to promise that if the suicidal depression regularly encompassing me does eventually get the better of me I will try to let you personally know where and when I plan for it to occur so that you can be close by to enable you to be the first in line to rifle through my pockets.

One thing that has become patently obvious to me in the past 12 months is that not everyone in the healthcare industry does actually care. Your first contact with me demanding money as opposed to asking after my welfare highlights that very point and is something that I have included in the book I am writing in an attempt to help young stroke survivors.

Yours sincerely
A Shaw

Copy to: Mr A Manktelow

Weather the Storm

My letter, which was written from the heart with emotion and real feeling, had the desired effect when about one week later, to the credit of the Park Hospital, I received a letter from the credit control department informing that they were to waive the outstanding amount as a 'gesture of goodwill'.

Furthermore, I received a letter from consultant orthopaedic surgeon Andrew Manktelow as follows:

Dear Andrew

I was devastated to receive your letter and accept your comments ….]. I have written directly to the credit control department at the park hospital about this and have enclosed a copy of my note for your information.

Whilst I was disappointed that the Hospital has chosen to chase you regarding the outstanding bill, my major concerns relate to your comments regarding your more recent depression and indeed suicide concerns. I was really desperately saddened to read this. I can fully appreciate the change in your level of activities now, compared to immediately prior to surgery, and the devastating effect this has had on you and all your family. As I have mentioned on the ... occasions we have met subsequently, there are parallels in our ages and indeed our young families. I fully empathise with your frustration.

I hope to have an opportunity to talk to you on the telephone in the not too distant future to discuss all this [and] I hope that our plans for further review of your hip are in place and that the Park Hospital will not bother you further with any concerns with bills.

I send you and your family my heartfelt best wishes.

Yours sincerely.

Mr. Manktelow's letter gave me a huge boost simply because throughout it said to me:

'Andy, I care about you and your situation'

Mr Manktelow's letter to the Credit Control department at the Park Hospital was copied to me and stated the following:

I have just read a very disappointing copy of a letter from one of my patients, Andrew Shaw, which he wrote to you on 31 January.

As Andrew has mentioned in his letter, he did indeed suffer a severe and debilitating stroke very soon after discharge following joint replacement surgery, which has had a very significant effect on him and his family

Clearly there is no reason for you to have been aware of his circumstances. I wonder if it would be best, with any similar long term unpaid bills, to contact my secretary, [name], in the first instance to ensure that there is no specific underlying reason before things are pursued further.

I will write directly to Andrew. We are now following him up at [alternative hospital] because, as he points out, he no longer has medical insurance as a consequence of him being made redundant

In the circumstances, I hope it will not be necessary to pursue things further although if there are any issues in this regard I should be grateful if you would discuss them with me. I would be prepared to make up any shortfall myself if necessary.

Please do not hesitate to contact me if you wish to discuss this further.

Mr. Manktelow's letter tells you all you need to know about him – he cares and thinks about people. In today's 'want everything and want it now' world he is a rare being and I owe him my gratitude. I feel honoured to have made his acquaintance. I would trust him with my life despite what happened.

In comparison to the wonderful Andrew Manktelow the healthcare industry also has its fair share of egos and persons who seem to have lost sight of the patient as priority number one. Toward the end of my stay in the DRI each and every therapist knew that I was desperate to try anything that might expedite my recovery. I've subsequently discovered that they knew of Patty Shelley and her excellent track record of helping stroke victims. For whatever reason no one thought to recommend Patty to me. The world of Physiotherapy seems to be a highly competitive spiteful women's world with each (Patty Shelley, Jan Jolly and Lou McBarnett excepted) keen to be the one credited with making the breakthrough! Indeed, both Patty and I gave Rose and Tracy the opportunity to attend one of her treatment sessions upon me and utilise the event as a teaching session. Rose declined which surprised me since Patty is a renowned international neurological specialist and, I think, probably the world's most renowned Bobath stroke rehabilitation tutor. Rose would have benefited from the free session but it became clear that NHS politics, rather than Rose herself, was the blocker. I'm surprised Rose didn't take up the opportunity to learn from the world's most admired and respected neurological physiotherapist. She might have picked up a little nugget of knowledge that could be beneficial to her other patients. Something got in the way of her attendance. Surely the wider spreading of Patty's knowledge and experience would be beneficial to all, patients and practitioners alike. Whilst ever politics is a factor in the world of physiotherapy and a key driver in NHS decision making the patient will suffer. I fear that the patient is not of paramount importance in the NHS.

> Knowledge Nugget– Be respectfully vociferous whilst listening to your instincts about what you need to recover. No one knows your body or how you feel better than you. Have your say but be guided, not ordered, by a good therapist.

Chapter Nine

The World of Physiotherapy

During my rehabilitative journey I encountered many different types of therapists. Physiotherapists, occupational therapists and speech therapists are the most important people in the fight to recover from the horrible effects of stroke. It seems to me that doctors have little, if any, influence in stroke recovery although they are key in prescribing the medication necessary to prevent or delay the onset of a further stroke or strokes. My own doctor, Richard Lodge, has been fantastic with me offering any help he could. I never like going to the surgery but I was always willing to make an exception to see the beautiful and understanding Dr Kathryn McGuiness. Fortunately for me I didn't need a speech therapist because even though my speech became 'jibberish' immediately during the onset of stroke it returned to normal within days. I found that fact quite reassuring in that I felt if my speech and eyesight could be affected and return then so could my finger and arm movement. I'm not sure of the medical facts supporting that but it seems logical to me.

Jan Jolly and Rose are good therapists and quite similar in application of techniques of therapy yet were very different in approach to Patty Shelley. In my view Patty has no equal in the world of physiotherapy. Rose and Jan supported my limbs as they took them through their range of movement in an attempt to re educate my brain and get muscles firing again. Patty did that too although to a much lesser degree. She also worked deep into my muscles with her fingers and thumbs to stimulate the motor 'pathways' whilst majoring on Bobath principles. On one occasion she worked around my left shoulder and then asked me to sit up and outstretch my arms. As if by magic (from 'magic hands' herself) I lifted my left arm and stretched out for the first time since the stroke. It was a wonderful moment and confirmed everything I had heard about and hoped for from Patty Shelley. Each time I left the Shelley Rehabilitation Centre I felt a little nearer to fitness and mobility, which was quite contrary to any NHS physiotherapy I had undergone. Patty shocked me when she said she thought my biggest problem was not the effects of stoke but a problem with my circulatory system. She then talked about the Autonomic nervous system and explained the root of my immobility might be due to an Autonomic system that had taken 'flight' after the trauma of a stroke leaving me with significant circulatory problems. Patty was the only therapist to ask me if I had noticed any coldness in body parts since the stroke. My left foot, knee and hand felt as though they had been refrigerated but I, incredibly, had not made the connection. Even though my knee was cold to the touch my upper and lower leg were warm and normal body temperature. I'm obviously not as in tune with my body as I think I am! I had noticed certain parts of my body were cold but knew nothing about the Autonomic Nervous System, so didn't consider the issue of much importance. Significantly, other than Patty, no one in the 'medical world' asked about or detected the 'coldness' problem. Nevertheless when Patty set to work on me I began to feel increased heat in the cold areas followed by increased feeling, sensation and movement. Unlike any other physiotherapy sessions with, Lisa Sewell, Rose or Jan after an hour with Patty I always noted a difference in movement, mobility and/or mood. During one session Patty worked upon my left foot, again getting deep into the tissue with her fingers and thumbs. After her manipulation my foot felt like it belonged to me for the first time since the stroke. The sole of the foot, which had been cold, soft and spongy, became warm, firm and sensitive. My walking was much improved thereafter and Patty said that once my left arm was operational I would be walking even better. Things began to look more promising that they had for a long time. I know Patty wanted me to get better just as much as I did and to experience her skill, professionalism and desire on my behalf was wonderfully encouraging and confidence giving. She has a special gift for dealing with the human body and her hands detect things that others couldn't. Patty, unlike other physios was constantly talking during treatment letting me know what she was doing and why whilst also asking for my input. However, never once did she make negative comment that I experienced from others. She would say 'I need to do something about your technique of going from sitting to standing because if we can get you driving more through your left leg it will help your shoulder stability'

That's quite different from saying 'Your sit to stand isn't right.' I felt with some physios their comments about what wasn't right rather than what needed to be done made me feel down. I was drowning and they were describing the water! Patty Shelley's approach seems to me to be just right! She doesn't describe the water she just throws a first rate life buoy within easy reach. Consequently I was keen to increase the frequency of visits to Patty's rehabilitation centre to hasten my recovery. I still hold the view that increased therapy frequency increases the rate of recovery although that view was discarded at the DRI. I'm keen to debate and question accepted wisdom but I realise where my limitations of knowledge are. Patty is, I think one of, if not, THE number one expert in Bobath treatment of stroke victims in a world where experts in such a discipline are few. 'Expertise' in any discipline is quite something and many who claim to be experts are not. I would argue they perhaps have a real interest and love in what they do. That doesn't qualify one as an expert. Patty Shelley is, however, an expert, her knowledge of Bobath is beyond all others in the world. On March 3 2006 Patty invited me to her practice to be filmed as a teaching model for her world wide teaching sessions. In attendance were two Japaneses students in Bobath principles. I learned a lot in the session as the students assessed me and verbally reported to Patty their observations and findings. It was dramatic when Patty said, 'Okay so if that's what you assess as the problem how can you change it?' To hear her say that encouraged me that immediate impacts were possible.

That students were prepared to fly to the UK from Japan to learn from Patty further highlighted my disappointment and dismay at NHS Politics that prevented physiotherapists learning from a great talent. The Japanese students travelled thousands of miles to work with and learn from Patty. NHS Politics would not allow therapists to visit Patty's practice just 30 minutes jog away. If such really is as I believe due to NHS politics rather than individual egos then it's a national disgrace and a tragedy and the stroke patient is the loser. To recover from stroke is difficult enough without the hindrance of egos and politics. That said, stroke recovery is possible.

Chapter Ten

Florida

On 21 July 2007 we set of from Manchester Airport to fly to Florida for a two week family break with our dear friends 'the Barbers' – Mark, Tracy, Jake and Sam.

The holiday went fantastically well even though I had to use my wheel chair most of the time due to the amount of ground we covered. We wanted to visit a number of the attractions and enjoy what they had to offer. Fortunately, the United States seems to be very proactive when it comes to providing for people with disabilities. I did everything I wanted to do and was able to participate as an equal. Mark, it seemed to me, spent most of his holiday pushing my wheelchair. I'd have much preferred to be walking but I enjoyed being so near to my friend as we were talking, laughing and joking constantly. The Florida attractions are easy to negotiate due to the care and attention put into wheel chair access. I was keen to join my friend in riding on the thrill rides that were there to be enjoyed. I soon realised that being in a wheelchair didn't necessarily mean being disadvantaged in such places. We were able to use wheelchair access to get to the front of the queuing hordes which is nice but is scant consolation for having wheels for legs. Despite the need for a wheelchair we did everything we wanted to do whilst also taking time to relax in the pool provided outside our holiday villa. During one relaxing moment in the pool Mark almost moved me to tears when he told me 'I think you've handled your situation really well pal and I'd like to think I could do the same if it ever happened to me'.

Stroke 8 Andy Shaw 10 (goal assist accredited to my friend Mark)

That's why I'm lucky to have him as a friend. One day in Universal's Islands of Adventure Mark, I, our wives and the children – Tom, Amy, Jake and Sam were gathered around a punch ball machine. Lots of young men and boys were awaiting their turn to demonstrate their manliness and testosterone. I couldn't resist, got out of my wheel chair and slowly limped into position as the ball was lowered down in front of me. Because of an inability to get a decent base of support and unsteady torso movement I barely tapped the ball and it hardly moved. I slumped back onto my wheels. Had the facility been available I'm sure the machine would have registered **'Weakling - sit down pussy !**' but I tried, at least I did that. On the final day of our holiday we went to an idyllic place called Wakiwa springs state park in Apopka. Again access was first rate even though there were some significant gradients to negotiate. Once again my good buddy was helping me get around by pushing the chair. As is the purpose of the park we hired a canoe and I tried to walk though the shallow water before climbing into our vessel. I found it very difficult to stand on one leg whilst trying to lift the other into the canoe until a lady staff member helped me. Mark was trying to pick up a paddle and at the same hold the boat still for me to clamber aboard. With enormous feeling and empathy the lady said to me 'What did you do to yourself honey ?'

When I told her she said 'my dad is disabled and I've got a big heart for people in your situation. We can look after you here and make sure you enjoy all we have to offer' Her attitude was a contrast to some of the attitudes I've encountered in Britain. I thanked her for her care, patience and sensitivity and said 'I'll see you next year when I can paddle for myself' Mark did a great job getting us smoothly up and down the river where we saw magnificent wildlife including crocodiles, alligators, turtles and fish. It was a wonderful day because of the companionship of my best friend, having my family with me, the fun and laughter we had, the wonderful sights we saw and the basic human warmth and consideration of the lady who helped me into the canoe. It's a wonderful life !

Stroke 8 Andy Shaw 11

The following day we began the long journey home having had a most magnificent holiday. Rather than a holiday it was more like two weeks of laughter therapy.

When we returned home I felt so bright, cheery and revitalised. I wanted to share my zest for life and feelings of well being so decided to write to hip surgeon Andrew Manktelow to tell him I was fine and doing just great. His reply gives a clear insight into the content of my letter. On 3 September 2007 he wrote:

Dear Andrew,

Many thanks for your letter. I am pleased to hear you are well mentally and there has been significant improvement in your physical situation. Specifically I was delighted to hear you have been on holiday to Florida and you have a new job. I was also pleased to hear your hip contiues to feel good. I am sorry I have not written to you after our last meeting in clinic. Life is always busy but I did have an opportunity to read the sections of your book, that you kindly left with me last time. I would hugely commend you in your efforts from this point of view. I have no doubts that your book will do well. It covers an extremely important area and your positive outlook and hard work will undoubtedly help and inspire others. I was moved very much by many of your experiences acutely around the time of the stroke, specifically relating to your family. Your motivation to protect them acutely particularly struck a cord (sic) with me relating to my own family. Your highlighted knowledge 'nuggets' are particularly important and I have taken the time to read through them. From my own point of view you are absolutely at liberty to write whatever you feel about me and my involvement in your story. (I note you suggested you would seek approval before it went to print, rest assured you have mine whatever you do or say.

The issue of why you had a stroke still burns me too. I continue to do a large number of join replacements in young and old patients. Joint replacement surgery remains, on the whole, a happy area in which to practise. My patients do well as they work hard to optimise their outcome and functional recovery. I have always tried to be supportive with patients who have not done quite as well as others. Thankfully though some might be slightly slower, the end result is almost uniformly good. Patients who have more sinister complications, such as infection or dislocation of their joints are 'burned indelibly' in my mind to ensure that I do everything possible to avoid complications. Similarly patients, such as yourself, who have unusual and devastating problems are always foremost in my mind. I have no specific thoughts as to why your stroke happened, the fact that it occurred so soon following major surgical intervention suggests some relationship, though this is not a situation I have seen previously or indeed subsequently within my own practise. Clots in the legs can and do occur despite prophylaxis. Very rarely these clots can progress to give lung clots, which can be of more sinister consequence. As I remember things in your situation, no clot was every (sic) demonstrated in your lung or indeed elsewhere. We have had long and detailed discussions before and I remain extremely disappointed I was not able to return you to the function I had hoped for when we ot rid of your hip pain. I remain inspired by your response to what happened acutely and indeed subsequently. I remain influenced by your situation in my professional and indeed personal life. I look forward to meeting you again in clinic. Please send my very best wishes to your wife and indeed the rest of your family. Please do not hesitate to contact me at Queens anytime to discuss things.

Yours sincerely Mr A R J Manktelow.

It is right and proper that Andrew finishes his letter using the word sincerely. I believe him to be a truly sincere fellow. I like him a lot.

Chapter Eleven

Exeter

Patty invited me to be a patient model at an advanced Bobath course at the Royal Devon and Exeter hospital where she was to lecture upon advanced techniques of the Bobath concept.

> Knowledge Nugget– The Bobath approach was pioneered and developed by Dr Karel and Mrs Berta Bobath. Begun in the 1940's the Bobath Concept is now well known and accepted in many countries as one of the leading approaches to encourage and increase the patient's ability to move and function in as normal a way as possible. More normal movements cannot be obtained if the patient stays in a few positions and moves in a limited or disordered way. The aim of the bobath approach is to help the patient to change abnormal postures and movements so that he or she is able to comfortably adapt to the environment and develop a better quality of functional skills.

Prior to the course I asked Patty what I might expect in the way of improvements by the end of the week. She told me that my walking should be improved. Although I was officially a patient on the course to be practiced upon by the attendees I opted, with Patty's approval to sit through the whole week and listen to the lectures delivered by Patty. She was truly inspirational and my confidence in her grew beyond the already elevated levels. My rationale was that if I could pick up some information, no matter how small, it might prompt my inquisitive mind to find a new recovery idea to explore.

> Knowledge Nugget– It's unreasonable to simply sit back and expect your therapist to fix you. You must do your bit whether that is to read and research, question or exercise. Your optimum effort is imperative for you to recover.

The week started with Patty welcoming the attendees and outlining how the week would be played out. She introduced me and my case as her patient and then I set to work giving a pre planned lecture entitlted 'Is Risk aversion damaging patient health care ? It was the first time I had lectured since the stroke and it went well. I felt confident, happy and assured.

The week which contained lectures and demonstrations was immensely interesting. I learned about brain cell plasticity and muscular alignment amongst other thought provoking subject areas. Each day the attendees had a patient, of which I was one, upon which to apply their newly learned skills. I was placed in the safe and skilled hands of Louise McBarnett from Stoke Mandeville Hospital's stroke rehab team and Yoshide Hokari, one of six Japanese students who had made the long journey to

England to learn from 'The Master' – Mrs Patty Shelly. Like Yoshi, Louise was great and not only is she a talented physiotherapist she could give Julia Roberts a run for her money in the beauty stakes !

I found it disturbing that the course would not have gone ahead without the Japanese attendees which is a sad reflection on the state of the UK's stroke patient care. I suppose I shouldn't have been surprised as months earlier Rose and her colleague Tracy at a Derbyshire hospital's physiotherapy had not been allowed to make the short journey across the small county to learn from Mrs Shelley. It's such a shame and disgrace that NHS politics or individual egos are so great that patient care is relegated to something other than the main priority. It's almost as though the hospital politicians are saying 'You're only a fucking patient and don't you ever forget it. You're here for us!

> Knowledge Nugget– It would appear that a multitude of things take precedence over the care of our fellow man including finance, politics and egos. Stroke care in the UK needs a shake up

Anyway, off I went to Exeter with my mum, dad and brother. It was like going back in time twenty five years to one of my wonderful childhood holidays in a caravan by the sea. and my emotional state improved so much because of it.

Patient's of some of the physios in attendance were present to be treated by the wonderful Mrs Shelley. Patty told them my story and at my request and with her approval I stayed around to listen when she said,

'Mr Shaw was referred to me by his Orthopaedic Surgeon on the 26th September 2006 A request was made for an assessment to ascertain the potential for future recovery

His present history includes a right hip resurfacing on 13/12/05

He suffered a left hemiplegia on 29/12/05

He has no past medical history of note

My assessment was that he has no mid line and has asymmetrical patterns and balance difficulties

His dressing and general ADL (Activities for daily living) needs assistance

He has no true selective movement in Left Upper Limb and has severe left shoulder pain

He has some selective movement of Left hip, knee and foot.

He also has autonomic symptoms. His skin is cold and clammy especially distally. He also has respiratory problems and temperature control problems along with sensory loss and a decrease in proprioception

Andy has mobility problems. His base of support is decreased along with a lack of dorsi flexion in his left foot. He also has emotional issues

He suffers with a weakness of right lower limb especially hip extensors and has an inability to stand on either leg with trunk control'

As I listened to the assessment the thing that raced through my mind was that all of this was as a result of a clot of blood finding its way to my brain. How could such a seemingly small clot cause such devastation?

I can only describe it as a car crash in the city centre at rush hour. Perhaps a small event but devastation, confusion and congestion all around the accident site.

Patty, with my prior approval also shared with the course attendees my list of frustrations and goals along with the improvements I felt I had made and what I had learned during my short time with her;

Frustration list

Inability to write whilst using the telephone.

Left arms lags when rolling over

Managing a broadsheet newspaper

Reading in the bath.

Dressing (slipping tie knot, driving left arm through a sleeve, putting on socks.)

Condition influences food selection ('spoon or fork friendly' meals only)

Improvements made under Mrs Shelley's care;

Significantly improved walking gait (speed and quality)

Increased control of left arm but no functional use as yet

Made a return to work.

Developed some finger movement and a pinch grip.

A significant reduction in fatigue.

An improvement in mental clarity and a reduction in 'fogginess'

Learned:

That the emotional and physical state are mutually dependent.

So much about the human body and its modus operandi that I was shocked by my own ignorance.

The effects on the body of the ANS.

Muscular alignment is critical to normal movement.

Confidence in one's therapist breeds emotional stability.

That no part of the functional body is independent from all other parts.

That the whole family has suffered from the effects of the stroke.

A positive outlook is helpful toward recovery and subsequently there is no room for negativity on a recovery road.

At the end of the week involving many lectures and practical demonstrations I was incredibly fatigued but mentally on top of the world. My walking had improved ten fold and I'd learned so much from a brilliant group of physiotherapists from across the UK and Japan. Lou McBarnett and Yoshi Hokari worked tirelessly for me and I shall always be grateful to them for their help, dedication and professionalism. To add to that there was also, of course, the inspirational and brilliant Mrs Shelley. All of the attendees seemed to hang on her every word and seemed to be in absolute awe of her talent. It seemed to me that the group's respect and gratitude for the mercurial Mrs Shelley knew no bounds.

Chapter Twelve

Two Years On

As I write this chapter on Saturday 29 December 2007 I'm exactly two years on from the day of the stroke. I'm walking pretty well to the point that it's not so noticeable that I've had a stroke.

Stroke 8 Andy Shaw 12

My left arm though still 'stuck' at the shoulder bends at the elbow and wrist very well. I do use it in everyday living. My left leg is responsive to all my brain's motor commands and my head does not feel fuzzy and stroke affected like it used to. I'm really in quite good shape considering the physical and emotional battering I've been subjected to over the last two years. The battering has been at the hands of a severe stroke, uncaring employers and insensitive people. Most important I feel that I'm still getting better which greatly contradicts popular medical opinion about stroke recovery. I've been told by medical *experts* that most recovery comes in the first nine months after the stroke but my experience tells me that is wrong. Organ plasticity is a wonderful thing and I know I'm still improving even now and I haven't done yet. I know that in time no one will ever know that I've been affected by this most devastating but beatable affliction. Stroke recovery has no definite and visible finish line and no one can tell you how much time you'll have to serve without each faculty (speech, sight, mobility) that you may have lost. Patience really will be a virtue. According to Wikipedia, patience is the ability to endure waiting, delay, or provocation without becoming annoyed or upset, or to persevere calmly when faced with difficulties. What it doesn't define is how soul destroying and frustrating it can be and the route back to fitness from ill health is a testing as anything I have ever known or experienced. One just has to sit tight and see it through and the rewards will come. Tough times don't last forever – weather the storm.

Stroke 8 Andy Shaw 13

It's not full time yet because I intend to continue my story to prove to the medical world that stroke recovery can continue years after the event. More than that I intend not just to beat stroke but to give it a bloody good hiding. Stroke is getting it's ass kicked big time by this fighter. I'm a human being, an Englishman, a husband, dad, brother and son and a Nottingham Forest supporter! I reckon I can whip most anything although I know something will eventually beat me and I know when when my last fighting day will be. Until then I'll keep kicking stroke up the butt!

Chapter Thirteen

Visualisation

I have used the practice of visualisation in my life on many occasions. Visualisation is a technique that develops the mind and body relationship to synergise to allow the power of the mind to help the body achieve a desired state. When I competed the in the Mr UK in 1991 and the Mr Britain body building championships at Wembley arena in 1994 I employed the power of my mind to assist my dietary and training efforts to develop the physique I'd imagined I should have when I walked out onto the stage to perform my routine. The fact that I didn't win didn't concern me at the time because I knew I'd achieved my desired state. In the months leading up to the competition I had visioned my physique and how it should look on the day. It came to fruition the way that I had visioned it. Of course the desired state has to be physically possible. If my disability was due to amputation then the power of the mind cannot grow new body parts. I'll leave that to the power of prayer even though that doesn't work. I got so desperate that I even tried that. I have no doubt that visualisation has been one factor in helping me achieve many things in my life I know it's worked for me and it can for anyone. The mind, like the brain is as yet I feel little understood. I seldom embark on anything important without having played out the event and its desired outcome in my mind before hand. People often say to me 'just imagine how you'll feel when you run and kick a ball again' and my response is simple 'It will feel just like I expected it to as I visioned it'. In simple terms I'm thinking myself better that's why I know I will beat the effects of this stroke. Whilst undergoing therapy at Patty's clinic one day she was stretching me out on the therapy plinth and said to me 'imagine you're swimming'. I got so locked into that mind set that when I opened my eyes Patty said 'Are you okay Andy? Her concern was that I had a look of amazement on my face and I knew why. Such was my mind so locked in to having a swim I was surprised I wasn't wet when I came back to real time! I'm slowly eating away at my goals and they've already been achieved in my visual imagery. I've refereed a children's soccer match in my mind. Soon I'll actually physically achieve it. You wouldn't bet against it would you ? That isn't half bad for an ordinary guy who not so long ago was cast out of the four limbed world and into his own one limb world with massive problems and an Everest sized mountain to climb !

In my experience, severe ill health causes one to try almost any avenue to search for a solution. Ultimately, with stroke or any condition beyond current medical scientific advances I feel that hard work, determination, a positive mind set and visualisation gives the best likelihood of recovery. Oh, and Patty Shelley too! I tried other things like reiki and acupuncture with limited effect and even got to the point of prayer which , I firmly believe is a waste of time and effort. It just doesn't work – pure and simple.

Chapter Fourteen

The World of Disability

The stroke entered me into a whole new world – the world of disability. Initially, because of the hip operation and stroke I had lost the use of both legs and one arm. A wheelchair became quite a fixture in my life in the months after the stroke. An unwanted fixture but a very necessary one although I knew that eventually I would be out of it making me much better off than some wheelchair users. I found life to be hard with wheels for legs although, unfortunately, the attitudes of some people make it harder still. I had countless negative experiences whilst using wheels as legs but utilised them as positives to fuel my recovery. Most of the negatives were encountered here in the United Kingdom – England. My worst experience was in the Derbyshire Restaurant in the DRI with the near 'does he take sugar' experience. Also at the DRI when trying to use the ATM cash point I was struggling to get close enough to read the screen when some probably well meaning but rude middle aged woman said to me. ' Are you going to be much longer because I'm in a hurry and I can go a lot faster than you', I replied with a curt ' I'm struggling to read the screen from here (seated) but I'm going as quick as I can !' There was nothing more said after that as an uncomfortable silence followed until I was told 'These machines aren't very good for people like you are they?' to which I replied ' People like me! why, what am I like?' She started to back pedal like a Derby County defender. I could have got her off the hook much quicker but I chose to let her squirm for a while until I eventually said "let me tell you how I happen to be in this chair' from where I went on to explain about the stroke. When I'd finished talking she said 'I find it very tragic' giving me the opportunity to straighten her out good and proper by saying ' It's not half as tragic as your attitude towards wheel chair users!'. The woman looked tearful so I thought if you're going to turn on the water works I'm out of here and off I went on my wheels for legs. I don't know for sure but I'll bet she had a restless night and will think about her future behaviour. Unfortunately her future strategy will probably be to avoid anyone with a visible disability. People seem to be uncomfortable around those with disability and with that particular lady I might just have made a difference. A small difference but a difference nevertheless.

The incident that was equally upsetting was as a result of being requested to do a speech on risk and safety by a professional conference organiser in London. They'd used me before as a guest speaker having a high profile in the discipline of risk and safety and in the airline industry. When I explained my new situation their interest in me cooled and when I asked why that was I was told 'It might be difficult to get you on stage and in front of the microphone without a lot of fuss and messing about'. To which I replied 'If you're ever putting on a conference about the Disability Discrimination Act I'd love to be a speaker at that. In fact I'll give you a special mention!' I put the phone down and heard nothing more. Fuck them!

I had the occasional humorous moment though. When parking adjacent to a disabled space in the local supermarket, a friend, walking by, who I'd not seen for ages thought I was in the disabled bay and shouted 'Shawy you wanker what's your fucking disability?' to which I replied 'Same as yours – tourettes - you thick twat now fuck off!' All good bloke's industrial humour.

> Knowledge Nugget– The medicine of laughter! Take copious amounts of it throughout day. Laughter releases positivity and a sense of well being.

I realise that I was probably very touchy and irritable whilst I was on wheels for legs and also whilst ever I was physically struggling with my walking and arm movement. At times I was a difficult man to reach as I turned my thinking in on myself with the sole aim of physical recovery. I wasn't altogether sure where my anger was coming from or aimed at but, once again, the brilliant Patty Shelley, gave me food for thought when she told me that according to Chinese medicine pressure on the liver creates anger. Was it that my slumped torso was creating pressure on my liver turning me into the hateful bastard that I seemed to have become? Sometimes it was impossible to win with me ! When I was invited to an awards evening by the Nottinghamshire Football Association having been nominated for 'Coach of the

Year', I didn't want to go and wouldn't have done so but for the insistence of my wife. Once I had begun walking a little better I resumed my coaching duties for a local girls soccer team. My coaching technique and ability was no better or worse that it had been pre stroke except that I could no longer physically demonstrate a skill as I once could. I felt that my nomination was because I was battling on despite a stroke and was disabled. I felt it was saying 'poor little Andy, he keeps trying even though he's disabled now'. Well, the award was for 'coach of the year' not 'sad case of the year'. I was relieved when I didn't win because I didn't deserve it and I don't want anything that I haven't earned. My friend Steve Pritchard, who has helped me in my efforts to become a successful coach won the award and I was genuinely delighted for him . He deserved it far more than me because he's a better coach than me (at the moment !) but I'm going to be a really first rate coach in the future (I know it because I've visioned it !) As my recovery has gathered pace allowing me to be much more mobile than in the early dark days immediately after the stroke I now feel I am in a very privileged position. I'm a fairly well able bodied individual with a real insight into the world of disability. You can only truly know the world of disability when you've experienced it. Maybe someone in authority will realise and let me work with passion on behalf of disabled people in the years to come. I'd like to make a difference because I know what it's like to choose a restaurant not because of its service and food standards but because of it's accessibility. I really do know. I know how it feels to be treated like a second class citizen because of wheels for legs. In addition to that, physical disability removes more choice than simply which building one can access. Some clothes were impossible for me to wear because of the types of fastenings etc. My food choice was influenced by having just one operational arm as I opted for meals that did not require cutting by knife. My favoured steak has been off the menu unless some kind soul accompanying me was willing to cut my meal up. I also found the looks of a waiter or waitress quite disconcerting if I was eating alone and ordering a steak but asking if it could be cut up for me. I suppose at initial viewing I look quite normal. I have two arms but one just doesn't operate and I have come to the conclusion that a disability that isn't obvious to the eye is, to many, not a disability at all. I was deeply hurt when a former business associate remonstrated with me about the clothes I was wearing at a seminar. I had arrived at the event minus a tie and in casual trousers. I did the best I could to look presentable and was hurt when a few weeks later he told me if I was going to dress like that not to bother coming again because the delegates wouldn't like it. It's pehaps a sign of the times – if you don't look 'right' then you aren't 'in' regardless of the reasons causing the disdain.

There is no doubt that the effects of stroke on my physical situation have been difficult to deal with. However, the emotional effects because of the actions of people have been, in many cases, as difficult to deal with perhaps because, with a little thought and consideration, the hurt could have been avoided. Is such because people don't care about those with a disability or, again, are we just living in a time where some just don't care about anyone but themselves!

Chapter Fifteen

The Final Word?

Strokes are devastating and whilst the effects of a stroke differ from person to person I sincerely believe that such devastation can be battled against so that a stroke doesn't have the biggest say on the life of its victim. I know many people who suffer strokes are not as fortunate as me because they are killed or devastated beyond the human capacity to mount a recovering reply. I certainly don't want to give the impression that anyone not recovering from a stroke lacks fight or will. It so happens that I've been able to fight back despite the severity of the stroke I had. Perhaps the next one, if and when it comes, will kill me outright or leave me cuckoo.

A I see it, life is a series of moments, some good some not so good. The stroke was a moment and I decided it was up to me to create a richness in my life despite being a stroke victim. There are many types of victim and I intended to be the type that got up, dusted myself down and fought on without making a big issue out of it. As I have previously said, I'm not just recovering from a stroke, I'm inspiring my children. I had moments pre stroke which I savour and I'm having moments post stroke which I'm enjoying equally . Despite the stroke I think I'm better placed now to enjoy life and all it has to offer than I ever was pre stroke. My life was on hold for a bit as I battled away day by day to win. Winning is a game of inches my friend Humphrey Walters told me. A penalty kick can stop on the line or just roll over it. A stroke affected arm can't reach the light switch one day but in time it makes it there ! Keep on keeping on ! Stroke recovery is certainly a marathon duration and marathons are never won or lost after a few paces.

It's certainly a slow process, but I seem to remember the tortoise won in the end. If you're young and enthusiastic but have had a stroke the sooner you realise that rehabilitation is a long, long road the better off you'll be. A victory is one thing but against stroke it's very much about how you win so you don't carry any residual physical disabilities. I'm winning, Chris Dent has won and so can you. Winning is everything and second is nowhere. Coming second against stroke is a heavy and costly defeat !

Andy is currently working on his second book 'Calm Seas' which continues his stroke rehabilitation story.

Chapter Sixteen

Chronology of Stroke

December 29 2005: Stroke occurred with loss of speech, perphiperal vision and left sided limb movement - immediate hospital admission

December 30 2005: transferred to Queens Medical Centre, Nottingham

January 2006: Transferred back to Derby Royal infirmary

February 06 2006: 42nd birthday

March 01 2006: Walked for the first time post stroke

March 30 2006: Discharged from hospital to home. Walked off the ward with the aid of a walking stick of stick. Left arm and hand still unresponsive

April 7 2006:	1st community physiotherapist visit to my home
April 2006:	Fell at home – unable to get to my feet. Contacted my nephew, Rob, by mobile phone who came to my aid.
April 2006:	Began outpatient physiotherapy with Rose at a Derbyshire NHS hospitl out patient physiotherapy department
May 01 2006:	Met Chris Dent for the first time
May 2006:	Flew to Holland for my daughter's soccer tournament
June12 2006:	Driving assessment – approved to drive an automatic transmission and steering adapted vehicle
July 2006:	Returned to work
July 28 2006:	left the UK for a 2-week holiday in Majorca
October 2006:	Made redundant from my role as Director of Risk and Safety at a UK Airline under the terms of a compromise agreement
December 02 2006:	First visit to Patty Shelley at the Shelley Rehabilitation Clinic

December 2006:	Slight improvement in range of left arm and thumb movement
December 29 2006:	1st anniversary of stroke occurrence
January 01 2007:	Purposely lay onto the floor to see if I could arise without assistance, which I did – Happy New Year!
June 2007:	Started to feel the stroke induced fatigue and mental dullness beginning to subside
July 2007:	Family holiday in Florida with our dear friends, the Barbers
September 2007:	Attended, via invitation,the Advanced Bobath course as a patient model at the Devon and Exeter Hospital in Exeter in the South West of England led by the brilliantly talented and gifted Mrs Patty Shelley.

Bibliography

Thurlow, BC (1981: 386) in , 'no soul to damn, no body to kick: an unscandalising inquiry into the problem of corporate punishment'

McCann. A Stroke Survivor:

Hicks. G, 2007, One Unknown, Rodal International Ltd, London

McCrum. R My Year Off:

Smits & Smits - Boone (1994)'Hand recovery after stroke' Butterworth Heinmann

Rowlands. A 2006: 6 in 'Stroke news Summer 2006 Volume 24.2' 'Working your way through a stroke'

Knight. F (2007) 'A stroke of genius' Yours Magazine issue 015 July 17 -30.

About the Author

Andrew (Andy) Shaw is a 44 years old married father of 2 living in Derbyshire, England. He is a highly qualified Risk Manager with many years experience in aviation having served bmi, EasyJet and First Choice. He has a Master's degree in Risk earned at the renowned Scarman Centre at Leicester University. He is a Director of the UK's Institute of Risk Management and at 41 years of age he survived a massive stroke which had a devastating effect on his life.

Andy is currently working on his second book *Calmer Waters* the sequel to *Weather the Storm*.

Andy can be contacted through AuthorHouse.

Printed in the United Kingdom by
Lightning Source UK Ltd., Milton Keynes
138368UK00001B/17/P